TABLE OF CONTENTS

Part 3. CLINICAL NURSING SKILLS

Basic Physical Care and Observation

Units **1-2**

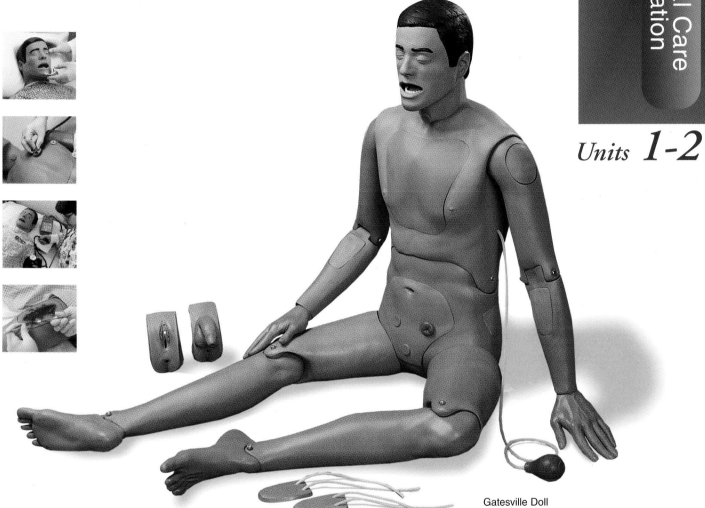

Gatesville Doll
GDW-2300

For information on MPL products call 1-800-433-5539

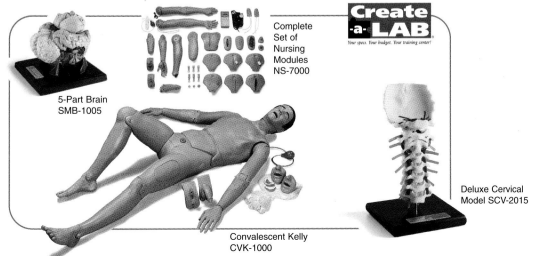

5-Part Brain
SMB-1005

Complete
Set of
Nursing
Modules
NS-7000

Create
-a- LAB
Your specs. Your budget. Your training center!

Convalescent Kelly
CVK-1000

Deluxe Cervical
Model SCV-2015

UNIT 1.   PROVIDING BASIC PHYSICAL CARE

1-1. BATHING / SKIN CARE / SAFETY

Learning Objectives

The learner is expected to:

1. Explain and demonstrate the special physical care required for older adults.

2. Perform and document an assessment of a surgical wound.

3. Describe precautions used during bathing for clients with selected health problems.

4. Analyze assessment data to determine priority nursing diagnoses.

5. Develop a plan of care for an older adult.

6. Define common terms associated with bathing and skin care.

Critical Thinking Skill Practice and Validation

- Explanation

- Interpretation

- Analysis

- Evaluation

- Self-regulation

Critical Thinking Activity 1-1-1

You are preparing to bathe a 75-year old woman who has a midline abdominal surgical incision that is open to air. She is receiving continuous oxygen via nasal cannula at 2L/min for chronic obstructive pulmonary disease (COPD). The client is usually alert and oriented, but has intermittent episodes of disorientation and confusion.

a.   Demonstrate the special skin care that this client requires during bathing. Why does her skin require special care? *

b.   During the client's AM care, what position should she be placed in and why? *

c.   If you need to leave her bedside, demonstrate what interventions you will provide before leaving her room. *

d. In the space below, identify at least two nursing diagnoses that are appropriate for this client. State at least one expected outcome for each diagnosis, including relevant outcome criteria. (Use the NOC system as a guide, if you are familiar with it.)

e. List appropriate nursing interventions that are needed to help the client meet her outcomes. (Use the NIC system interventions and activities, if you are familiar with them.)

f. What information about the client's abdomen is important to observe? What should you report to the nurse? *

g. Assess the client's abdomen. Document your findings here and have another student, or your instructor, check your note for feedback.

* These activities and questions are also appropriate for unlicensed personnel, such as nursing assistants and patient care technicians.

Critical Thinking Activity 1-1-2

While assisting with a partial bath, you prepare to wash a client's legs and back. The client was recently admitted to the hospital with a large deep vein thrombosis (DVT) in her left lower extremity (LLE) and is receiving continuous IV heparin via an infusion pump.

a. What special precautions will you take when bathing the affected leg and why? *

b. The client tells you that she has very dry skin on her feet. What nursing interventions should you implement? *

c. Demonstrate how to help the client change into a clean gown. *

* These activities and questions are also appropriate for unlicensed personnel, such as nursing assistants and patient care technicians.

Critical Thinking Activity 1-1-3

One of your home care agency's aides calls to report that her male client has recently become incontinent of urine. She asks you what she should do and reminds you that her client is uncircumcised.

a. What is the desired outcome for this incontinent client? (Use the NOC system as a guide, if you are familiar with it.)

b. What preventive actions should you recommend for the client's skin care at this time? *

c. Demonstrate how to provide perineal care for an uncircumcised man. What special precaution should you take? *

* These activities and questions are also appropriate for unlicensed personnel, such as nursing assistants and patient care technicians.

7

Review of Terms 1-1-4

Match the term in the left column with its definition from the right column.

___ 1. Jaundice

___ 2. Pallor

___ 3. Ecchymosis

___ 4. Erythema

___ 5. Lesion

___ 6. Petechiae

___ 7. Purpura

___ 8. Blanching

___ 9. Edema

___ 10. Thrush

A. Reddish, purple area of the skin

B. Redness of the skin

C. Whitish hue to an area of the skin

D. Fungus infection (yeast) of the mouth

E. Yellowish appearance of the skin

F. An area of broken skin

G. Excess fluid in the tissues

H. Pinpoint reddish spots on the skin

I. Paleness; absence of color

J. Bruising

8

Learning Objectives

The learner is expected to:

1.   Explain how to dress a client who has hemiparesis (one-sided weakness) and maintain a safe environment.

2.   Perform and document an assessment of the oral cavity.

3.   Demonstrate oral hygiene for a comatose client.

4.   Demonstrate how to wash a client's hair while the client is in bed.

Critical Thinking Skill Practice and Validation

- Explanation

- Analysis

- Inference

- Self-regulation

Critical Thinking Activity 1-2-1

A 60-year old man is admitted for rehabilitation following a left brain attack (stroke). He has right-sided hemiparesis (weakness) and expressive aphasia (inability to speak). As part of his rehabilitation, the client is learning how to perform activities of daily living (ADLs). Yesterday, he fell in the Physical Therapy Department while walking with his quad cane, but he was not injured.

a.   Demonstrate how you would teach the client to put on a shirt that buttons down the front. What principle should you keep in mind when teaching dressing techniques to a client with hemiparesis? *

b.   How will you determine if the client understands your instructions, as he has aphasia? *

c.   What interventions should you initiate to help prevent further falls for the client? (Use the NIC system interventions and activities, if you are familiar with them.) *

* These activities and questions are also appropriate for unlicensed personnel, such as nursing assistants and patient care technicians.

Critical Thinking Activity 1-2-2

A 67-year old woman was struck by a car three weeks ago and has been in a coma since that time. The client has a gastrostomy tube for feedings and a Foley catheter to continuous drainage.

a. Demonstrate how to remove the client's dentures and provide good oral hygiene. Clean her dentures and then place them into her mouth. *

b. What assessments should you perform related to her oral cavity? Document your findings here and have another student, or your instructor, check your note for feedback.

c. Demonstrate one way to wash the client's hair in bed. *

* These activities and questions are also appropriate for unlicensed personnel, such as nursing assistants and patient care technicians.

1-3. POSITIONING / MOBILITY SKILLS

Learning Objectives

The learner is expected to:

1. Use correct body mechanics when positioning and moving clients in bed, when transferring a client from the bed to a chair, and when transferring a client from the bed to a stretcher.

2. Determine if assistance is needed when positioning and moving clients.

3. Identify observations that are needed when transferring clients.

4. Make an occupied bed for a post-trauma client.

Critical Thinking Skill Practice and Validation

- Analysis

- Inference

- Evaluation

- Self-regulation

Critical Thinking Activity 1-3-1

A 15-year old client has been admitted to the pediatric unit with multiple left leg fractures, right radial fracture, and tissue trauma as a result of an ATV (all-terrain vehicle) accident. He is 5'8" and weighs 180 pounds. A trapeze and overhead (Balkan) frame has been added to his bed to assist in mobility.

a. Demonstrate how you should move the client up towards the head of the bed. How would you determine if you need assistance to move him? Be sure to use good body mechanics while moving the client. *

b. Position the client on his right side, using pillows and other support devices to maintain this position. *

c. What outcomes are expected for this client? (Use the NOC system as a guide. if you are familiar with it.)

d.   What are two ways that you could make an occupied bed for this client? Demonstrate one of these two methods. *

Critical Thinking Activity 1-3-2

A 6'2" client weighing 250 pounds has just returned to your surgical unit from the post-anesthesia care unit (PACU) following a lumbar laminectomy and spinal fusion of L_2 - L_5 vertebrae. The surgeon's orders read: "Logroll pt. Q2h until tomorrow AM. OOB to chair in AM with lumbar orthotic device."

a. Demonstrate how you should move the client this evening. Should you obtain assistance to turn him? Why or why not? *

b. Assess his surgical dressing and document your findings below. Have another student, or your instructor, check your note for feedback. What unusual assessment findings should be reported immediately to the surgeon?

c. Demonstrate how to get the client OOB to a chair and vice versa. What observations should you make when getting him up for the first time? What is the purpose of the orthotic device? Will you need assistance to transfer him? Why or why not? *

d. The client is scheduled for a lumbar spine x-ray. Demonstrate how you should transfer him to a stretcher. Will you need assistance? Why or why not? *

Critical Thinking Activity 1-3-3

You are assigned to a 45-year old client who had a craniotomy. She is alert, oriented, and able to communicate, but tends to be impulsive when transferring or using her walker. She is weak in her right leg and foot, but otherwise has good muscle strength.

a. Demonstrate how you would teach the client to transfer from the bed to the wheelchair with your assistance.

b. Ask a fellow student to simulate this client's condition. Using a gait transfer belt, assist the student while he or she ambulates with a walker. What principle will you use to assist the student? *

c. How will you teach the client to ambulate when she progresses to a cane? On what side of the body should the cane be placed? How high should the cane be for safety and support of the client?

* These activities and questions are also appropriate for unlicensed personnel, such as nursing assistants and patient care technicians.

1-4. FEEDING

Learning Objectives

The learner is expected to:

1. Demonstrate how to feed a client who requires total care.

2. Identify special considerations for feeding a visually impaired client.

3. Explain the need for special considerations when feeding a client with impaired swallowing.

4. Develop a plan of care for a client with dysphagia (difficulty swallowing)

Critical Thinking Skill Practice and Validation

- Analysis

- Inference

- Explanation

- Evaluation

Critical Thinking Activity 1-4-1

A young male client sustained a traumatic brain injury (TBI) and cervical spinal cord injury and is quadriplegic (paralyzed from the neck down). He has a Halo jacket with cervical traction in place. He is unable to perform any activities of living (ADLs) at this time. You are assigned to care for him today.

a.   What position should you place the client in for feeding and why? *

b.   Demonstrate how you would feed him. *

c.   If he gets food lodged into his airway and requires the Heimlich maneuver, show how you would perform this maneuver.

d. What outcomes are expected for this client related to feeding and nutrition? (Use the NOC system as a guide, if you are familiar with it.)

* These activities and questions are also appropriate for unlicensed personnel, such as nursing assistants and patient care technicians.

Critical Thinking Activity 1-4-2

An older adult in the nursing home where you work has recently begun experiencing dysphagia due to advanced esophageal cancer. She requires assistance with her meals because she wears glasses for poor vision from bilateral cataracts. The resident is alert and oriented, but is becoming increasingly depressed as a result of her declining health.

a. Position this client in preparation for mealtime. *

b. To help the client feed herself, how should you set up her tray and why? *

c. What outcomes are desired for this client related to feeding and nutrition? (Use the NOC system as a guide, if you are familiar with it.)

d. What types of food would most likely be better tolerated by the client?

e. List interventions for this client that would help meet the desired outcomes listed in c. (Use the NIC interventions and activities, if you are familiar with them.)

* These activities and questions are also appropriate for unlicensed personnel, such as nursing assistants and patient care technicians.

22

1-5. ELIMINATION / INTAKE AND OUTPUT

Learning Objectives

The learner is expected to:

1. Explain appropriate options for assisting a hip surgery client to meet elimination needs.

2. Demonstrate how to assist a hip surgery client with meeting elimination needs.

3. Interpret intake and output results and take action as needed.

Critical Thinking Skill Practice and Validation

- Explanation

- Interpretation

- Inference

- Evaluation

- Self-regulation

Critical Thinking Activity 1-5-1

An older adult had an open reduction/internal fixation (ORIF) of her left hip yesterday. She tells you that she needs to urinate as soon as possible. Her Foley catheter was discontinued this morning, and she has not voided since it was removed.

a. What desired outcomes related to her hip surgery should you keep in mind while assisting the client with her elimination needs? (Use the NOC system as a guide, if you are familiar with it.)

b. What special precautions should you take to help her meet the above identified, desired outcomes? *

c. What options do you have to assist the client with meeting her elimination needs? Demonstrate one of these options. *

d. What action, if any, should you take if the client is unable to void? *

Critical Thinking Activity 1-5-2

A middle-aged client has been admitted to the special care unit with a diagnosis of lower gastrointestinal (GI) bleeding. She is receiving a full liquid diet and a continuous IV infusion of 5%D/0.45NS at 125 mL/h. The client has a Foley catheter in place for strict intake and output monitoring.

a. Which of the following foods/liquids are allowed on a full liquid diet? *
    (Check each one that applies.)

___Coffee   ___Cottage cheese   ___Soda (pop)   ___Pudding

___Broth   ___Orange juice   ___Cold cereal   ___Jell-O

b. For breakfast, the client drank 3/4 of a carton of milk, 4 ounces of apple juice, and about a fourth of her hot tea. She also had a half glass of water with her morning medications. What is the client's total intake for this morning in mL? Show your work here and have a student or instructor check your work for feedback. *

c. What laboratory values should you monitor for a client with GI bleeding?

d. At the end of your 8-hour shift, the patient care tech (PCT) reports that the client's total urinary output is 190 mL for the past 8 hours. What actions, if any, should you take? Why or why not?

1-6. PHYSICAL RESTRAINTS

Learning Objectives

The learner is expected to:

1. Apply several types of physical restraints (infant and adult).

2. Determine appropriate alternatives to physical restraints for adults.

3. Identify the least restrictive types of physical restraints.

4. Explain nursing responsibilities when caring for clients who are physically restrained.

5. Determine which nursing responsibilities related to care of clients in restraints could be **delegated** to unlicensed nursing personnel.

Critical Thinking Skill Practice and Validation

*   Analysis

*   Inference

*   Evaluation

Critical Thinking Activity 1-6-1

A six-month old infant has been admitted to the pediatric unit with severe gastroenteritis and dehydration. In preparation for starting intravenous therapy, you apply a mummy restraint.

a. Demonstrate how to apply a mummy restraint. You may either use a mummy board or bath blanket. *

b. What nursing responsibilities are important while caring for the infant who is restrained?

c. How long should the infant be restrained?

d. What outcomes are desired for this infant? (Use the NOC system as a guide, if you are familiar with it.)

* These activities and questions are also appropriate for unlicensed personnel, such as nursing assistants and patient care technicians.

30

Critical Thinking Activity 1-6-2

You are assigned to care for a middle-aged adult who has a history of alcoholism and cirrhosis of the liver. His liver enzymes are very high, and he has become disoriented, confused, and sometimes combative as a result. The client has a nasogastric (NG) tube in place, but has pulled it out three times in the past two days.

a.   What alternatives to physical restraints might you implement? Will the health care setting make a difference in the alternatives you select? Why or why not? *

b.   If physical restraints are used for this client, which type would be the most appropriate and <u>least</u> restrictive? Apply this type of restraint to the client while he is sitting in a chair. *

c. In the space below, develop a plan of care for this client who is physically restrained. Include nursing diagnoses, expected outcomes and nursing interventions. (Use the NIC interventions and activities, and the NOC system as a guide, if you are familiar with them.) For each intervention, indicate which ones could be **delegated** to unlicensed nursing personnel.

* These activities and questions are also appropriate for unlicensed personnel, such as nursing assistants and patient care technicians.

32

Hammond, M. & Levine, J.M. (1999). Bedrails: Choosing the best alternative. *Geriatric Nursing, 20*(6), pp. 297-301.

This excellent article challenges the notion that bedrails (siderails) keep clients safe. In the long-term care setting, bedrails are classified as physical restraints and health care professionals must find alternatives to their use if possible. The authors provide a client assessment guide to determine if bedrails can be removed, and a list of devices and other alternatives that can be implemented in place of bedrails.

Mayhew, P.A., et al. (1999). Restraint reduction: Research utilization and case study with cognitive impairment. *Geriatric Nursing, 20*(6), pp. 305-308.

The authors describe how they used research findings to implement a restraint reduction program for their cognitively impaired clients in a veterans' health care system. Over a two-year period, the facility's restraint rate decreased by 28%. The authors also noted that restrained clients require more nursing time than unrestrained clients due to the monitoring and related care. Thus, restraint reduction saved nursing time.

UNIT 2. ASSESSING VITAL SIGNS

Learning Objectives

The learner is expected to:

1. Demonstrate how to take temperature of infants and children using several methods.

2. Convert Celsius temperatures into Fahrenheit and vice versa.

3. Identify strategies for managing fever in pediatric and adult clients.

4. Describe physiologic changes in older adults that affect temperature.

Critical Thinking Skill Practice and Validation

- Interpretation

- Analysis

- Inference

- Self-regulation

Critical Thinking Activity 2-1-1

A four-year old boy who has an earache and fever is being seen in the office by the pediatric nurse practitioner (PNP). You prepare to take his temperature using a mercury-in-glass thermometer because the electronic thermometer is not working. The child begins to cry and is afraid that having his temperature taken will "hurt."

a. What method would be best for taking his temperature with the glass thermometer? Why? Demonstrate this procedure. *

b. What strategies should you use to reassure the child that he will not experience discomfort during the procedure? *

c. The client's temperature is 103.2 degrees F. What is his temperature using the Celsius measurement scale? Show your work here and have another student, or your instructor, check it for feedback.

d. What interventions will you suggest to the child's mother to manage his fever? (Use the NIC interventions and activities, if you are familiar with them.)

* These activities and questions are also appropriate for unlicensed personnel, such as nursing assistants and patient care technicians.

Critical Thinking Activity 2-1-2

You have been asked to take a temperature on a 77-year old nursing home resident using the infrared tympanic thermometer (ITT).

a. What are the advantages of this type of thermometer? What are the disadvantages and precautions? Demonstrate the use of this type of thermometer if available. If it is not available, use an electronic oral thermometer. *

b. The client's temperature is 36 degrees C. What is her temperature using the Fahrenheit measurement scale? Show your work here and have another student, or your instructor, check it for feedback.

c. Is the temperature obtained in b. (above) within the expected range? Why or why not?

*These activities and questions are also appropriate for unlicensed personnel, such as nursing and medical assistants, and patient care technicians.

Critical Thinking Activity 2-1-3

Read the annotations for the Suggested Readings at the end of this unit. What conclusion could you draw regarding the best method for taking temperature in very young and older adults? How did you come to that conclusion?

Learning Objectives

The learner is expected to:

1. Determine important pulses to monitor in selected clinical situations for adults and infants.

2. Explain when **delegating** vital signs may not be appropriate.

3. Interpret pulse values and compare with expected ranges.

4. Define common terms associated with taking pulse and respirations.

Critical Thinking Skill Practice and Validation

- Interpretation

- Explanation

- Inference

- Analysis

Critical Thinking Activity 2-2-1

You are caring for a diabetic client who just returned from having a right femoral arteriogram. She has a history of severe peripheral vascular disease (PVD) and hypertension. Last year, the client had a left below-the-knee amputation (BKA).

a.   Which pulses should you monitor carefully following this invasive procedure and why?

b.   Should monitoring this client's pulses be **delegated** to an unlicensed assistive staff member? Why or why not?

c.   If her pulses are not palpable, what actions should you take and why?

d.   What is the relationship between diabetes mellitus and peripheral vascular disease?

Critical Thinking Activity 2-2-2

You prepare to take a pulse on a newborn as part of a perinatal home visit in the Healthy Start program. The infant is crying and the new mother seems very anxious and distraught.

a. Which pulse should you take to ensure an accurate measurement? Should you take the pulse while the child is crying? Why or why not?

b. The infant's pulse rate is 200 bpm. Is this value within the expected range for the infant's age?

c. What effect might the infant's crying and mother's anxiety have on the infant's vital signs, if any? Explain your answer.

Critical Thinking Activity 2-2-3

An older adult is admitted to the telemetry unit with acute congestive heart failure, dysrhythmias, and uncontrolled hypertension. She is complaining of shortness of breath and has pitting edema in both feet. Her breath sounds indicate crackles at the bases of both lungs.

a.   When you take her radial pulse, what might you anticipate regarding the quantity and quality of her pulse? *

c.   You decide to also take an apical pulse and find that it is 102 bpm. Her radial pulse is 84 bpm. Why is there a difference between her radial and apical pulses? What is this difference called?

d.   What changes in her respirations might you expect as a result of her medical diagnosis and adventitious breath sounds?

*These activities and questions are also appropriate for unlicensed personnel, such as nursing and medical assistants, and patient care technicians.

Review of Terms 2-2-4

Match the term in the left column with its definition from the right column.

____1. Bradycardia   A. Increased heart rate above 100 bpm for an adult

____2. Cheyne-Stokes   B. Alternating periods of apnea, decreased respirations, and increased respirations

____3. Biot's   C. No respirations

____4. Kussmaul's   D. Regular strong pulse followed by regular weak pulse (every other beat is strong)

____5. Tachycardia   E. Decreased respirations below 12 per minute for an adult

____6. Pulsus paradoxus   F. Decreased heart rate below 60 bpm for an adult

____7. Apnea   G. Rapid and deep respiratory pattern

____8. Bradypnea   H. Increased respirations above 20 per minute for an adult

____9. Pulsus alterans   I. Slow and deep or rapid and shallow respiratory pattern, followed by apnea

____10. Tachypnea   J. Regular pulse, then decrease in pulse amplitude associated with respirations

2-3. BLOOD PRESSURE

Learning Objectives

The learner is expected to:

1.   Analyze assessment data to determine interventions related to obtaining accurate blood pressure measurement.

2.   Identify special needs of clients that could affect blood pressure measurement.

3.   Document relevant data related to client blood pressure.

4.   Interpret blood pressure values to determine if they are in the expected range.

Critical Thinking Skill Practice and Validation

*   Interpretation

*   Analysis

*   Inference

*   Self-regulation

*   Evaluation

Critical Thinking Activity 2-3-1

You are assigned to care for an older woman in a nursing home who is 4'11" tall and weighs 95 pounds. She has a long history of osteoporosis and arthritis, and is weak on her left side from Parkinson's disease. You prepare to take her blood pressure.

a. What precautions will you take to ensure that you get an accurate blood pressure reading? *

b. While taking her blood pressure, she tells you that she sometimes gets dizzy. In the space below, write a note to document her concern and the actions you would implement. Have another student, or your instructor, check your note for feedback.

c. What priority nursing diagnosis is appropriate for this client? What outcome(s) is (are) desired? (Use the NOC system as a guide, if you are familiar with it.)

d. When taking her blood pressure, you have difficulty hearing it. What actions should you take at this time? *

Critical Thinking Activity 2-3-2

You are assigned to a middle-aged client who has been diagnosed with pneumonia and possible tuberculosis. She is receiving continuous intravenous fluids in her right arm and has a history of a left simple mastectomy (no removal of lymph nodes).

a.   When taking the client's blood pressure, what assessment data should you consider in deciding how to perform the procedure. Why? *

b.   What options do you have in deciding where to take the blood pressure? Which site is preferred and why? *

c.   The blood pressure reading is 154/92. Is this measurement within the expected range for an adult? What actions should you take at this time? *

*These activities and questions are also appropriate for unlicensed personnel, such as nursing and medical assistants, and patient care technicians.

2-4. PAIN: THE FIFTH VITAL SIGN

Learning Objectives

The learner is expected to:

1. Assess and interpret acute and chronic pain in adults and children accurately and completely.

2. Identify options for acute and chronic pain management.

3. Determine which option represents best practice for pain management for selected clients.

Critical Thinking Skill Practice and Validation

- Interpretation

- Analysis

- Inference

- Self-regulation

Critical Thinking Activity 2-4-1

You are assigned to care for several clients today on an orthopedic unit. One of your clients is a man who had his left knee replaced two days ago. His PCA pump was discontinued this morning and he has just returned from Physical Therapy for rehabilitation, including strengthening exercises and ambulation in the parallel bars. He tells you that his surgical leg muscles are having spasms that are "quite uncomfortable."

a.   What is the first action that you should take? Why? Describe how you will carry out this action.

b.   The client tells you that his pain feels like a 5 on a 0 to10 pain scale. What does this mean? Would you expect that a client having acute pain might have vital sign changes? Why or why not?

c.   What options do you have for managing his pain? How will you decide which option to use?

Critical Thinking Activity 2-4-2

You are caring for a 22-month old toddler in the pediatric oncology unit. She has acute lymphocytic leukemia (ALL) and is receiving chemotherapy. You find her crying in the corner of her crib. When you touch her she cries louder and you suspect that she may be in pain.

a.   What other observations might you make to determine if the child is having pain?

b.   Will her vital signs be altered by chronic malignant pain? Why or why not?

c.   If you determine that she is having pain, how might you measure its intensity?

d.   What options for pain management do you have?

e.   In the space below, write a note that addresses the client's behavior, your assessment, and the option(s) for managing pain that you chose.

Acello. B. (2000). Meeting the JCAHO standards for pain control. *Nursing2000, 30*(3), pp. 52-54.

This article describes the new standards for all health care agencies that are accredited by the Joint Commission on Accreditation of Healthcare Agencies (JCAHO). These standards focus on both pain assessment and management for all clients across the life span.

Fallis, W.M. (2000). Oral measurement of temperature in orally intubated critical care patients: State-of-the-science review. *American Journal of Critical Care, 9*(5), 334-343.

This article summarized the results of 10 studies found in the literature about the best method for taking temperature in clients who are intubated with an endotracheal tube. Many nurses take temperature rectally, resulting in embarrassment, increased stress for clients, and increased use of resources. including time. The results of the reviewed studies showed that the oral method is valid for clients who are intubated.

McConnell, E.A. (2000). Using a Doppler device. *Nursing2000. 30*(7). pp. 17.

This one-page photo guide illustrates a step-by-step procedure for using a Doppler ultrasound device when a pulse is not palpable. This device is an important assessment tool for nurses caring for clients with vascular health problems.

Prentice, D. & Moreland, J. (1999). A comparison of infrared ear thermometry with electronic predictive thermometry in a geriatric setting. *Geriatric Nursing, 20*(6), pp. 314-317.

This study compared the accuracy and reliability of three methods for measuring temperature among older adults, using an infrared tympanic thermometer, oral electronic thermometer, and oral glass thermometer. The glass thermometer readings were found to be the most reliable, followed by those from the electronic thermometer and tympanic thermometer. Larger samples need to be used for follow-up studies before these results can be generalized.

Sganga, A., et al. (2000). A measurement of four methods of newborn temperature measurement. *MCN: American Journal of Maternal-Child Nursing, 25*(2), 76-79.

The researchers compared four methods for taking temperature in newborns, using the glass thermometer, electronic thermometer, tympanic thermometer, and digital thermometer. Athough the tympanic thermometer was cost-effective, it was not sensitive and specific, and did not correlate well with the glass thermometer readings. The authors concluded that the use of tympanic thermometers is not a good choice for healthy newborns.

Stuppy, D.J. (1998). The Faces Pain Scale: Reliability and validity with mature adults. *Applied Nursing Research, 11*(2), pp. 84-89.

The researchers used the Faces Pain Scale-- originally used to assess pain intensity in children-- to evaluate the tool's use with older adults. The tool was found to be a reliable and valid tool for this population as well. For clients who cannot verbally communicate, the tool would help to assess pain intensity in that group.

Physical Assessment

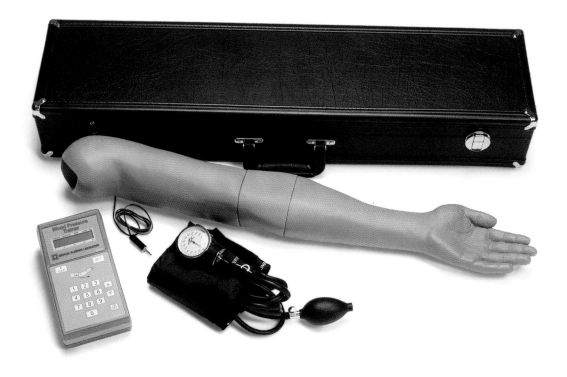

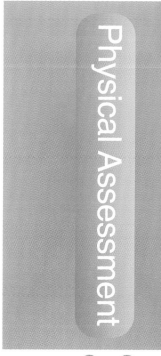

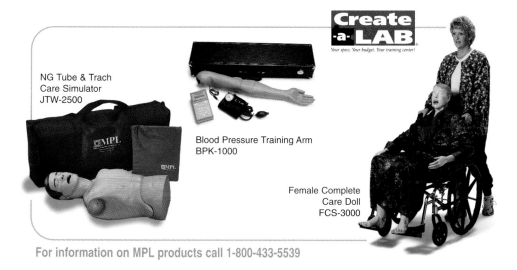

Create -a- LAB
Your specs. Your budget. Your training center!

NG Tube & Trach
Care Simulator
JTW-2500

Blood Pressure Training Arm
BPK-1000

Female Complete
Care Doll
FCS-3000

UNIT 3. CARDIOVASCULAR AND RESPIRATORY ASSESSMENT

3-1.   Peripheral Vascular Assessment

3-2.   Heart and Breath Sounds

Suggested Readings

Learning Objectives

The learner is expected to:

1. Explain the differences in physical assessment findings for clients who have arterial and venous insufficiency.

2. Demonstrate how to perform and document a lower extremity assessment.

3. Determine desired outcomes for clients with cardiovascular problems.

4. Identify desired outcomes for a client with ascites due to cirrhosis of the liver.

5. Explain the significance of edema as part of fluid balance assessment.

6. Interpret findings associated with peripheral pulse assessment.

Critical Thinking Skill Practice and Validation

*   Explanation

*   Interpretation

*   Evaluation

*   Self-regulation

Critical Thinking Activity 3-1-1

A middle-aged adult comes to the medical clinic with complaints of bilateral leg cramping, which worsens with walking, cold feet, and decreased sensation and numbness in both feet, especially on the soles of the feet. The client has a history of Type II diabetes mellitus, diabetic neuropathy, and peripheral vascular disease.

a. What other physical assessment should you perform? Do you think her symptoms are more commonly associated with peripheral arterial disease or venous disease? Why?

b. Describe the differences between physical assessment findings common in clients with peripheral arterial insufficiency and those with peripheral venous insufficiency. Make a table to show the differences.

c.   Should you test for the Homan's sign? Why or why not?

d.   Demonstrate a thorough peripheral extremity assessment and document your findings. Feel free to add information that might be present in your assessment of this client. Have another student, or your instructor, check your note for feedback.

Critical Thinking Activity 3-1-2

An older adult is admitted to the medical unit with a diagnosis of cirrhosis of the liver and heart failure. He has severe ascites and pitting edema in both ankles. His breathing is labored and he is irritable and drowsy.

a. When you read the physician's admission history and physical examination report, you note that the client has 1+ pedal pulses bilaterally. What does this notation mean?

b. What other peripheral pulses should you assess?

c. What pathophysiology explains the client's ascites and ankle edema?

d. How should you assess the amount of edema that the client has? Does this finding reflect an accurate assessment of fluid balance in the body? Why or why not?

e. What desired outcomes are realistic for this client? (Use the NOC system as a guide, if you are familiar with it.)

f. What is the best way to assess fluid balance in the body? Demonstrate this procedure using the equipment you have available. (You may use a fellow student, if preferred, to demonstrate this skill.) *

*These activities and questions are also appropriate for unlicensed personnel, such as nursing and medical assistants, and patient care technicians.

3-2. HEART AND BREATH SOUNDS

Learning Objectives

The learner is expected to:

1. Perform and document heart and lung sounds.

2. Interpret common adventitious breath sounds.

3. Develop a plan of care for a client with congestive heart failure.

4. Define common terms associated with cardiopulmonary assessment.

Critical Thinking Skill Practice and Validation

- Interpretation

- Explanation

- Inference

- Analysis

- Evaluation

- Self-regulation

Critical Thinking Activity 3-2-1

You are assigned to care for a young man who has had his first myocardial infarction. He has been very healthy until this event, and is extremely anxious about his future, including how coronary artery disease will affect his lifestyle.

a. When performing a cardiac assessment, where would you expect to locate his point of maximal impulse (PMI)? Find his PMI and take an apical pulse.

b. Listen for heart sounds at the base and apex of his heart. Where is the base of the heart located? Where is the apex? What heart sounds do you hear and where are they heard the loudest?

c. Listen to his breath sounds. Where do you hear tracheal sounds? Where do you hear bronchial sounds? Where do you hear vesicular sounds? Does this client have any adventitious breath sounds?

d. In the space below, write a note to document your findings related to heart and breath sounds. Have another student, or your instructor, check your note for feedback.

e. What might you tell the client to help alleviate his anxiety about the MI?

Critical Thinking Activity 3-2-2

A 9-year old child is admitted to the pediatric unit with acute asthma and an upper respiratory infection. On admission, you prepare to do a thorough history and physical assessment.

a.   What questions about the diagnosis should you ask the client or parent/guardian? *

b.   When you listen to the client's breath sounds, what adventitious breath sounds would you expect to hear and why? Listen to the child's breath sounds and document your findings in the space below. Have another student, or your instructor, check your note for feedback.

c.   What principles of medical management will be used to treat this child and why?

*These activities and questions are also appropriate for unlicensed personnel, including nursing and medical assistants and patient care technicians.

Critical Thinking Activity 3-2-3

An older nursing home resident has a history of congestive heart failure, stroke, and hypertension. She usually requires minimal assistance with her activities of daily living (ADLs), but today is very lethargic, "short of breath," and anorexic. She refuses to get out of bed and becomes agitated when the nursing assistant tries to help her with AM care.

a. What assessment should you perform for the client at this time and why? Perform the assessment and document your findings in the space below. Have another student, or your instructor, check your note for feedback.

b. As part of her assessment, you note adventitious breath sounds in her left lung. What sounds do you hear? Are they consistent with her suspected diagnosis? Why does a client with congestive heart failure often have these lung sounds?

c. Identify two priority nursing diagnoses for this client and determine desired outcomes for each. What interventions are appropriate for her to meet the desired outcomes? (Use the NIC interventions and activities and the NOC system as a guide, if you are familiar with them.)

Review of Terms 3-2-4

Match the term in the left column with its definition from the right column.

_____ 1. Crackles

_____ 2. Murmur

_____ 3. Rubor

_____ 4. Hypoxia

_____ 5. Wheezes

_____ 6. Fremitus

_____ 7. Retraction

_____ 8. Tripod position

_____ 9. Orthopnea

_____ 10. Bruit

A. Deep-reddish skin color

B. Upright position for breathing

C. Adventitious breath sound caused by narrowing of airways

D. Drawn-in neck and chest muscles, usually indicating airway obstruction

E. Swooshing sound heard over a narrowed artery

F. Adventitious breath sound heard in alveoli due to fluid or alveolar opening

G. Swooshing sound caused by turbulent blood flow in the heart or great vessels

H. Lack of oxygen in the blood

I. Client leaning forward with arms braced against knees, chair, or bed

J. Vibrations felt on chest wall

Ludwig, L.M. (1998). Cardiovascular assessment for home healthcare nurses. Part II. Assessing blood pressure and cardiac function. *Home Healthcare Nurse, 16*(8), s547-554.

This article describes assessment techniques to obtain an accurate blood pressure, as well as heart and lung sounds. Medication management and documentation for home care is also discussed.

O'Hanlon-Nichols, T. (1998). Basic assessment series: The adult pulmonary system. *American Journal of Nursing, 98*(2), 39-45.

The author continues the series of articles that review physical assessment of each body system. In this article, the procedure for a complete respiratory assessment is reviewed, including an emphasis on normal and adventitious breath sounds.

Owen, A. (1998). Respiratory assessment revisited. *Nursing 98, 28*(4), pp. 48-49.

The author reviews respiratory assessment with an emphasis on auscultation for normal and adventitious breath sounds as they relate to common respiratory diseases.

UNIT 4. NEUROLOGIC, SENSORY, AND MUSCULOSKELETAL ASSESSMENT

4-1. LEVEL OF CONSCIOUSNESS AND MENTAL STATUS ASSESSMENT

Learning Objectives

The learner is expected to:

1.   Identify the most important aspect of the neurologic assessment.

2.   Interpret Glasgow Coma Scale results.

3.   Perform a mental status assessment.

4.   Develop a plan of care for a client with early dementia.

Critical Thinking Skill Practice and Validation

- Interpretation

- Analysis

- Evaluation

- Inference

Critical Thinking Activity 4-1-1

An older client is hospitalized for bladder suspension surgery and is admitted to your surgical unit for postoperative care. The client has a Foley catheter, a PCA (patient-controlled analgesia) pump, and continuous intravenous fluid infusion. On arrival to the unit postoperatively, it was noted by the day nurse that the client was alert and oriented. During her first night on the unit, however, she got out of bed to go to the bathroom without using her call light and subsequently fell. You find her lying on the floor near the bathroom door. Her arm is oozing blood because her IV dislodged, and her catheter is out as well. She is conscious and tells you that she hit her head on the foot of the bed when she fell.

a.   What assessment will you perform first and why?

b.   On initial post-fall assessment, you find that her Glasgow Coma Scale (GCS) score is 15. What does this score mean? What interventions are appropriate for the client with a score of 15 on the GCS?

c.   The next day, the client's GCS decreases to 12 (3 for "Best Eye Opening Response," 5 for "Best Motor Response," and 4 for "Best Verbal Response"). Should you take any further action at this time? Why or why not?

Critical Thinking Activity 4-1-2

You are visiting a client in the home for the first time. She is 77 years old and lives with her younger sister in a small apartment on the first floor. The client was discharged from the hospital following an episode of hypoglycemia (related to diabetes mellitus), hyponatremia (low serum sodium), and hypokalemia (low serum potassium). She has been on Cardizem and Dyazide for several years for treatment of hypertension and dysrhythmias. When interviewing the client, you note that she has poor short-term memory, but can recall life events that occurred when she was a child. Her sister states that she has been having this problem for several years, and that it seems to be getting worse. She also mentions that the client walked out of the home two nights ago and could not recall how to return to the house.

a.   What questions should you ask the client to determine her mental status? *

b.   What formal tools could you use to do this assessment?

c.   What priority nursing diagnoses are appropriate for this client? What outcomes are realistic for her? What interventions might you suggest to the sister to help meet the desired outcomes? (Use the NIC interventions and activities and the NOC system as a guide, if you are familiar with them.)

*These activities and questions are also appropriate for unlicensed personnel, such as nursing and medical assistants, and patient care technicians.

Learning Objectives

The learner is expected to:

1. Perform and document the quick neurologic assessment, also called "neuro checks."

2. Determine priority nursing diagnoses and/or collaborative problems and desired outcomes for the postoperative craniotomy client.

3. Determine priority nursing diagnoses and/or collaborative problems and desired outcomes for the post-stroke client.

Critical Thinking Skill Practice and Validation

- Analysis

- Evaluation

- Self-regulation

Critical Thinking Activity 4-2-1

A 10-year old child is transferred from the neurosurgical step-down unit to the pediatric surgical unit. She had a craniotomy for removal of a large benign brain tumor, but is medically and neurologically stable. The surgeon's orders include performing "neuro checks" every 4 hours while she is awake. The client tells you that she is worried that the students in her 6th grade class will make fun of her hair where it has been shaved.

a.   What does a "neuro check" include in most health care agencies?

b.   Perform a "neuro check" on this client. In the space below, document your findings. Have another student, or your instructor, check your note for feedback.

c.   Determine her priority nursing diagnoses and/or collaborative problems and desired outcomes for each. (Use the NOC system as a guide, if you are familiar with it.)

Critical Thinking Activity 4-2-2

A middle-aged adult is admitted to the Emergency Department with complaints of a severe headache, weakness on the left side, and numbness in the left lower leg. On initial assessment, the client was able to answer questions appropriately and had no problems with speech. After being in the ED for several hours, though, his condition changed and he became aphasic and lethargic. He was admitted to the medical unit.

a.   When you assess the client on admission to the medical unit, you note that his face droops and he is unable to move his left arm and leg. What further assessment is required for him at this time? Perform this assessment.

b.   What members of the interdisciplinary team will be involved in his care and why?

c.   Develop a plan of care for this client that includes three nursing diagnoses, desired outcomes, and interventions. (Use the NIC interventions and activities and NOC system as a guide if you are familiar with them.)

4-3. EYE AND EAR ASSESSMENT

Learning Objectives

The learner is expected to:

1.   Identify common physiologic changes of the eye associated with aging.

2.   Perform an assessment of the eye and ear.

3.   Develop a plan of care for the infant with otitis media.

Critical Thinking Skill Practice and Validation

•   Analysis

•   Inference

•   Evaluation

•   Self-regulation

Critical Thinking Activity 4-3-1

You are caring for an older resident in the nursing home who complains that her glasses must need changing because she is having problems seeing. She also complains that her vision is blurred and that she sometimes "sees two" of everything.

a.   What questions might you ask her to get more information about the history of her vision problem? *

b.   When you look carefully at her eyes, you notice that her pupils seem to be white rather than black, as expected. The left pupil is whiter and larger than the right pupil. What problem do you think she may have based on this observation? What other physical assessment should you perform at this time? Perform the eye and vision assessment.

*These activities and questions are also appropriate for unlicensed personnel, such as nursing and medical assistants, and patient care technicians.

Critical Thinking Activity 4-3-2

A parent brings her infant daughter to the clinic with a fever and constant crying. She tells you that the child has been pulling on her right ear since last night, and that there was drainage on the crib sheet this morning near the head of her bed.

a.   What physical assessment should you perform on the infant at this time and why? Perform this assessment and document your findings. Feel free to add information that is consistent with the child's probable diagnosis. Have another student, or your instructor, check your note for feedback.

b.   Develop a plan of care for the infant, including at least two priority nursing diagnoses and expected outcomes. Include nursing interventions to help meet these outcomes in your plan. (Use the NIC interventions and activities and the NOC system as a guide, if you are familiar with them.)

Learning Objectives

The learner is expected to:

1. Interpret findings from assessment of the spine and joints.

2. Perform a musculoskeletal assessment and document findings.

3. Identify desired outcomes for the client with rheumatoid arthritis.

4. Explain the major differences between osteoarthritis (degenerative joint disease) and rheumatoid arthritis.

5. Define common terms associated with musculoskeletal assessment.

Critical Thinking Skill Practice and Validation:

- Interpretation

- Explanation

- Analysis

- Inference

- Evaluation

- Self-regulation

Critical Thinking Activity 4-4-1

You are the office nurse for a local pediatrician. As part of your role, you perform a screening physical assessment for every infant and child who comes to the office. Today, a young mother brings her 2-month old boy in for a well-baby checkup.

a.   When performing a musculoskeletal assessment on this baby, what observations and techniques should you perform?

b.   What congenital musculoskeletal problems are common in this age group?

c.   Perform a musculoskeletal assessment on the infant and document your findings in the space below. Have another student, or your instructor, check your note for feedback.

Critical Thinking Activity 4-4-2

You are the nurse at a middle school and are planning the screening tests for the students for next year. One of the most important screenings for this group is scoliosis testing.

a.   What is scoliosis and how does it differ from kyphosis?

b.   Demonstrate how to screen for scoliosis in a pre-adolescent child and document your findings.

c.   If you find a child with possible scoliosis, what action should you take and why?

Critical Thinking Activity 4-4-3

A 68-year old woman who lives alone was diagnosed with rheumatoid arthritis when she turned 60. Her mother had the disease at an earlier age, and eventually became dependent due to severe pain and deformity. The client is afraid that she, too, will become dependent, and complains to you that she is in constant pain, especially in the morning when she suffers severe joint stiffness. The client also has a history of Type II diabetes mellitus and depression.

a. What other history questions should you ask her at this time? (Remember how to perform a comprehensive pain assessment.)

b. Perform a musculoskeletal assessment on this client.

c. What other physical assessment would be appropriate for this client in view of her medical diagnosis? What laboratory tests might be ordered for her at this time?

d.   Develop an interdisciplinary plan of care for this client, including priority nursing diagnoses, expected outcomes, and interventions. (Use the NIC interventions and activities and the NOC system as a guide, if you are familiar with them.)

e.   Compare and contrast the physical assessment findings of the client with rheumatoid arthritis and the client with osteoarthritis. Make a table to show the similarities and differences.

Review of Terms 4-4-4

Match the term in the left column with its definition from the right column.

___1. Kyphosis

A. A way to determine the presence of carpal tunnel syndrome

___2. Scoliosis

B. Hard, bony enlargements on distal finger joints

___3. Heberden's nodes

C. An audible grating sound that occurs when joints are moved

___4. Synovitis

D. A lateral deviation of the vertebral spine

___5. Genu valgum

E. A lateral deviation of the hand

___6. Phalen's test

F. Inflammation of the joint lining

___7. Subcutaneous nodules

G. A forward deviation of the vertebral spine

___8. Ulnar deviation

H. "Knock-kneed"

___9. Subluxation

I. Soft tissue enlargements that are common near joints

__10. Crepitation

J. Partial dislocation of the joint

Alexander, M. & Kuo, K.N. (1997). Musculoskeletal assessment of the newborn. *Orthopaedic Nursing, 16*(1), pp. 21-31.

This comprehensive article describes the components of the musculoskeletal assessment, including a concise history, complete developmental assessment, and thorough physical examination. The article can be used as a continuing education opportunity and there is a quiz at the end.

O'Hanlon-Nichols, T. (1998). Basic assessment series: A review of the adult musculoskeletal system. *American Journal of Nursing, 98*(6), 48-52.

The author continues the series on basic physical assessment by including ways to assess for sports injuries, such as sprains and strains, as well as carpal tunnel syndrome. Observation and palpation techniques help to determine the presence of any musculoskeletal health problems.

O'Hanlon-Nichols, T. (1999). Neurologic assessment. *American Journal of Nursing, 99*(6), 44-50.

The components of a basic neurologic assessment are described, including how to assess for mental status, cerebellar function, and cranial nerve problems. This article is a continuation of a series of articles that the author has written for the journal over the previous year.

UNIT 5. NUTRITIONAL AND ABDOMINAL ASSESSMENT

5-1. Nutritional Assessment

5-2. Abdominal Assessment

Suggested Readings

5-1. NUTRITIONAL ASSESSMENT

Learning Objectives

The learner is expected to:

1. Explain the key components of a nutritional assessment.

2. Interpret laboratory data related to nutrition and hydration.

3. Develop an interdisciplinary plan of care for a client who has inadequate nutrition and hydration.

4. Interview an adolescent who has a possible eating disorder.

5. Identify physical indicators of inadequate nutrition.

Critical Thinking Skill Practice and Validation

- Interpretation

- Analysis

- Evaluation

- Inference

- Explanation

Critical Thinking Activity 5-1-1

You are a home care nurse who is following an older woman for care of a large Stage IV pressure ulcer. She has been tube fed for two months, has advanced dementia, and is totally dependent in activities of daily living (ADLs). Her daughters, one of whom is a nurse, have been caring for her. Last week at her physician's office, the client's weight was 14 pounds less than her weight four weeks ago. Her significant laboratory data include:

BUN   87 mg/dL
Na   152 mEq/L
K   5.4 mEq/L

a.   What questions should you ask the caregiver at this time and why?

b.   What physical assessment should you perform at this time? Demonstrate this assessment.

c.   What is the significance of the laboratory results above? Are there other laboratory tests that should be performed at this time? If so, what might they include?

d.   What nursing diagnoses are appropriate for this client? What desired
        outcomes are realistic for her? (Use the NOC system as a guide, if you are
        familiar with it.)

e.   What interventions will help the client meet the desired outcomes? What
        members of the interdisciplinary team will you need to collaborate with and
        why? (Use the NIC interventions and activities as a guide, if you are
        familiar with them.)

Critical Thinking Activity 5-1-2

A 12-year old girl is brought to the pediatric nurse practitioner's office by her mother because the child has a very low food intake. The client is 5' and weighs 75 pounds. At her last annual examination visit, she was 4'11" and weighed 85 pounds. When you ask the client why she is not eating, she tells you that she is too fat.

a. What other questions should you ask the child and mother to complete a history? Should you interview them together or separately? Why? Pretend a fellow student is the client and interview her now. Record the answers below.

b. What are some of the physical indicators of inadequate nutrition? What physical assessment should you perform at this time and why?

5-2. ABDOMINAL ASSESSMENT

Learning Objectives

The learner is expected to:

1. Perform an abdominal assessment for an adult and infant.

2. Interpret abnormal abdominal assessment findings.

3. Plan culturally sensitive interventions for clients with abnormal assessment findings.

4. Define common terms associated with the gastrointestinal system and nutritional state.

Critical Thinking Skill Practice and Validation

- Interpretation

- Analysis

- Explanation

- Inference

- Self-regulation

Critical Thinking Activity 5-2-1

A certified nursing assistant in the nursing unit where you work reports that one of her older residents has a "swollen" abdomen. She tells you that the resident has had a poor appetite for the past two days, and is continuously oozing small amounts of liquid stool.

a. Demonstrate the physical assessment you should perform at this time.

b. What changes might you expect when listening to her bowel sounds?

c. Write a note to document your findings. (Assume that the client has bowel sounds that are consistent with small bowel obstruction.) Have another student, or your instructor, check your note for feedback.

d. What action should you take if you suspect that the resident has a bowel obstruction?

Critical Thinking Activity 5-2-2

A mother brings her 2-week old son to the ED with complaints of severe projectile vomiting and constant crying after taking his formula. She states that the infant's abdomen gets bigger after feeding. She also tells you that she went to her folk healer when the problem began two days ago, but the herbs she has given the baby have not worked.

a.   What other questions should you ask to complete the health history?

b.   What physical assessment should you perform? Demonstrate this assessment now.

c.   What actions should you take at this time and why? How will you incorporate the mother's cultural beliefs into your plan of care?

Review of Terms 5-2-3

Match the term in the left column with its definition from the right column.

___1. Obesity   A. An indicator of total body fat

___2. Body mass index   B. Protein-calorie malnutrition

___3. Serum albumin   C. A type of visceral protein

___4. Serum transferrin   D. Skin resistance indicating
                                   hydration

___5. Prealbumin   E. Liver enlargement

___6. Marasmus   F. Silvery white marks on the
                                   skin

___7. Skin turgor   G. A transport protein for
                                   thyroxine (T_4)

___8. Striae   H. More than 20% overweight

___9. Hepatomegaly   I. Protrusion of part of an organ
                                   through a body cavity wall

__10. Hernia   J. A sensitive indicator of body
                                   protein that can be measured or
                                   calculated

SUGGESTED READINGS

Berry, J.K. & Braunschweig, C.A. (1998). Nutritional assessment of the critically ill patient. *Critical Care Nursing Quarterly, 21*(3), pp. 33-46.

Bedside techniques for nutritional assessment are outlined in this article. Identifying clients at risk for undernutrition and providing nutritional support decreases medical complications and promotes early discharge from the critical care unit. The authors also discuss general guidelines for nutritional support.

Dudek, S.G. (2000). Malnutrition in hospitals. Who's assessing what patients eat? *American Journal of Nursing, 100*(4), 36-42.

This article describes the undernutrition and protein-energy malnutrition that is often overlooked while clients are hospitalized. The nurse has a responsibility to include nutritional assessment as part of the comprehensive physical client assessment. Older adults are especially at risk for nutritional health problems.

Hammond, K. (1999). Nutrition-focused physical assessment. *Home Healthcare Nurse, 17*(6), pp. 354-355.

The author advocates that home care nurses should include nutritional assessment into their home visits to promote better client outcomes. Much of this assessment can be obtained through a thorough health history.

UNIT 6.   URINARY AND REPRODUCTIVE ASSESSMENT

6-1.   Urinary Assessment

6-2.   Reproductive Assessment

Suggested Readings

6-1. URINARY ASSESSMENT

Learning Objectives

The learner is expected to:

1. Interpret abnormal findings related to urinary elimination.

2. Perform a dipstick urinalysis for screening urinary health problems.

3. Explain how cultural beliefs can influence a client's health care.

4. Identify appropriate nursing diagnoses and expected outcomes for a client with urinary stress incontinence.

5. Document health teaching for a client with stress incontinence.

Critical Thinking Skill Practice and Validation

- Interpretation

- Analysis

- Inference

- Self-regulation

- Explanation

- Evaluation

Critical Thinking Activity 6-1-1

An older man is scheduled for his annual physical examination with the internist. During his interview, he tells you that he has been having "trouble passing his water" for the past two months. He experiences no pain during urination.

a.   What questions should you ask him to complete a genitourinary history? *

b.   What laboratory testing might the physician order for this client and why? What physical examination techniques will the physician use?

c.   Perform an abdominal assessment on this client. What should you be checking for?

* These activities and questions are also appropriate for unlicensed personnel, such as nursing and medical assistants, and patient care technicians.

104

Critical Thinking Activity 6-1-2

A young Latino woman married last week presents in the Emergency Department with complaints of severe burning on urination, urinary frequency, and low-grade fever. She has been drinking cold liquids and avoiding spicy foods since her symptoms began, but these measures have not helped relieve her discomfort.

a.   What questions should you ask her to complete a health history? *

b.   When you obtain a urine specimen from her, you note that it has a strong odor, is very cloudy, and contains mucous threads and sediment. Perform a dipstick urinalysis on this sample. What do you expect to find?

c.   Explain how you plan to incorporate her beliefs about health interventions (hot/cold theory) into her plan of care.

*These activities and questions are also appropriate for unlicensed personnel, such as nursing and medical assistants, and patient care technicians.

Critical Thinking Activity 6-1-3

A middle-aged woman reports to her gynecologist that she has started having problems with bladder control, especially when she coughs, sneezes, or exercises. She wears sanitary pads for the dribbling, but feels embarrassed by the situation. She states that she has had six children, all by normal vaginal delivery.

a. What nursing diagnoses and expected outcomes are appropriate for this client? (Use the NOC system as a guide, if you are familiar with it.)

b. Teach the client what interventions may help her with her urinary health problem. Document your teaching in the space below.

6-2. REPRODUCTIVE ASSESSMENT

Learning Objectives

The learner is expected to:

1.   Explain how cultural beliefs influence client reproductive health.

2.   Perform a breast examination on an adult woman.

3.   Complete a reproductive health history.

4.   Teach breast self-examination (BSE) and testicular self-examination (TSE).

5.   Plan a teaching plan for clients with selected reproductive health problems.

6.   Define common terms associated with genitourinary assessment.

Critical Thinking Skill Practice and Validation

-   Explanation

-   Analysis

-   Inference

-   Self-regulation

Critical Thinking Activity 6-2-1

A young Asian American woman brings her middle-aged mother to the family nurse practitioner's office for a physical examination. The daughter tells you that her mother has not had a "female checkup" since the birth of her last child 20 years ago. The client told her daughter several days ago that she has a visible lump in her left breast. The client did not want to be seen by a health care provider, but came at the insistence of her daughter.

a. What questions should you ask her to complete the reproductive health history? *

b. What cultural beliefs may have influenced her reluctance to see a health care provider?

c. Perform a breast examination on this client and document your findings. Have another student, or your instructor, check your note for feedback.

d. What teaching does this client need?

*These activities and questions are also appropriate for unlicensed personnel, such as nursing and medical assistants, and patient care technicians.

Critical Thinking Activity 6-2-2

A young student goes to the college health center with complaint of a urethral discharge. He is very concerned that he may have testicular cancer. One of his friends was recently diagnosed with this problem.

a.   What questions should you ask to complete a reproductive history?*

b.   What teaching does the student need regarding sexually transmitted disease and testicular cancer?

c.   What psychosocial support should you offer him at this time?

*These activities and questions are also appropriate for unlicensed personnel, such as nursing and medical assistants, and patient care technicians.

Review of Terms 6-2-3

Match the term in the left column with its definition from the right column.

___1. Stress incontinence

A. Test to detect cervical cancer

___2. Urinary retention

B. Test to detect breast cancer

___3. Benign prostatic hyperplasia

C. Dribbling of urine when abdominal pressure increases

___4. Sexually transmitted disease

D. Nonmalignant enlarged prostate gland

___5. Urge incontinence

E. Involuntary control of bladder due to weak pelvic floor muscles

___6. Pap smear

F. Inability to empty the bladder

___7. Kegel exercises

G. Intervention for strengthening pelvic floor muscles

___8. Overflow incontinence

H. Test to detect prostate cancer

___9. Prostate-specific antigen

I. Dribbling of urine due to an overfilled bladder

__10. Mammography

J. Health problem resulting from sexual intercourse with an infected individual

Appleby, S. (1999). Stress urinary incontinence: Issues and answers for women. *Ostomy and Wound Management, 45*(1), pp. 50-53.

Since 1992 when the federal guidelines for adult urinary incontinence were published, there has been an increased focus on evaluation and management of incontinence. This article focuses on various options available to manage stress incontinence, one of the most common types of urinary incontinence among middle-aged and older women.

Klingman, L. (1999). Assessing the female reproductive system. *American Journal of Nursing, 99*(8), 37-43.

This comprehensive article describes how to perform a nursing assessment of the female reproductive system, including the reproductive history and physical examination. The author also discusses common diseases of the breast and genitalia.

Sneddon, D. (1999). Continence assessment in long-term care. *Professional Nurse, 15*(1), pp. 32-34.

The author describes the inappropriately diagnosed and managed urinary and fecal incontinence of clients in long-term care settings. All residents should have a complete continence assessment so that treatment can be initiated. Many types of incontinence are reversible and curable.

UNIT 7. SKIN ASSESSMENT

7-1. PRESSURE ULCER PREVENTION AND ASSESSMENT

Learning Objectives

The learner is expected to:

1. Assess pressure ulcers and document findings.

2. Interpret a client's risk of developing a pressure ulcer using the Braden scale.

3. Plan interdisciplinary interventions to help prevent nosocomial pressure ulcers.

4. Determine which pressure ulcer prevention interventions can be **delegated** to unlicensed nursing personnel.

Critical Thinking Skill Practice and Validation

- Interpretation

- Inference

- Self-regulation

- Evaluation

Critical Thinking Activity 7-1-1

An older adult is admitted to the nursing home for rehabilitation following a total knee replacement. According to the dietitian, his admission weight is below ideal body weight (IBW). His wife reports that he has lost "a lot" of weight during the past six months and his appetite has been poor. On admission assessment, you note that he is incontinent of urine at times and wears an external condom catheter. A small piece of Duoderm® covers a Stage II pressure ulcer on his sacrum that measures 1.5 cm X 1.0 cm.

a.   The client's Braden scale score on admission is 11. What does this score indicate about his risk for developing additional pressure ulcers?

b.   What preventive and management measures are needed for the client at this time? (Use the NIC interventions and activities, if you are familiar with them.) Can any of these interventions be **delegated** to unlicensed nursing personnel? *

c.   One of the nursing assistants tells you that she massages all reddened skin areas as she was taught in her aide class 15 years ago. How should you respond to her comment? *

d.   What members of the interdisciplinary team should you collaborate with to plan care for this client and why?

Critical Thinking Activity 7-1-2

A middle-aged paraplegic client is transferred from the Behavioral Health unit (admitted for severe depression) to the Medical unit for management of his atrial fibrillation and debridement of a Stage IV gluteal pressure ulcer. He continues to be followed by his psychiatrist and behavioral health case manager.

a.   Assess his pressure ulcer and document the findings in the space below. Have another student, or your instructor, check your note for feedback.

b.   What health teaching will the client need before he is discharged?

Learning Objectives

The learner is expected to:

1. Perform and document a comprehensive wound assessment.

2. Provide health teaching for a diabetic client who has a wound.

3. Plan emergency care for the client who experiences wound dehiscence.

4. Define common terms associated with skin and wound assessment.

Critical Thinking Skill Practice and Validation

- Analysis

- Inference

- Self-regulation

- Explanation

Critical Thinking Activity 7-2-1

You are an occupational health nurse working for a large manufacturing firm. After returning from a two-week vacation, an employee comes to your office and asks you to check his thigh wound. He states that he injured his leg while on the job last week. He has been caring for his wound at home. You note on his chart that he is a Type II diabetic.

a. Perform the wound assessment and document your findings below. Have another student, or your instructor, check your note for feedback.

b. What concerns do you have related to his soft tissue injury and diabetes mellitus and why? Does his wound need further treatment to facilitate healing? What health teaching should you provide?

Critical Thinking Activity 7-2-2

You have been assigned to care for an obese client who recently had abdominal surgery for a bowel resection. The nursing assistant reports that the client is very concerned about how her incision looks today. When you assess the client, you find that the incision has dehisced (opened).

a.   What assessment should you perform at this time?

b.   What action should you take at this time?

c.   Write a note to describe this experience, including wound assessment and your interventions. Have another student or your instructor check your note for feedback.

Review of Terms 7-2-3

Match the term in the left column with its definition from the right column.

___1. Dehiscence   A. Removal of dead tissue

___2. Evisceration   B. Inflammation and infection of skin and underlying tissues

___3. Gangrene   C. Unplanned opening (gaping) of an incision

___4. Eschar   D. Healthy, new tissue growth

___5. Necrosis   E. Blackened tissue caused by lack of blood supply

___6. Nosocomial   F. Leathery, black slough on a wound, such as a burn

___7. Debridement   G. Spilling out of abdominal contents through an open wound

___8. Granulation   H. Hospital or health care facility-acquired

___9. Cellulitis   I. Nonviable (dead) tissue

__10. Ulcer   J. A sore or skin lesion

SUGGESTED READINGS

Bergstrom, N., et al. (1998). Predicting pressure ulcer risk. *Nursing Research, 47*(5), pp. 261-269.

The authors used the Braden scale to determine its effectiveness in predicting high-risk clients in two tertiary care hospitals, two Veterans Administration Medical Centers, and two skilled nursing facilities for a total of 843 subjects. The tool was found to be a valid and reliable predictor of clients who would most likely develop nosocomial pressure ulcers.

Graff, M.K., Bryant, J., & Beinlich, N. (1999). Preventing heel breakdown. *Orthopaedic Nursing, 19*(5), pp. 63-69.

The authors stress the common occurrence of heel pressure ulcers among clients who have musculoskeletal health problems. Nurses must identify clients at high risk, especially those with immobility, advanced age, confusion, chronic illness, inadequate nutrition, and hip surgery. This article also describes appropriate preventive strategies.

U.S. Department of Health and Human Services. (1992). *Pressure ulcers in adults: Prediction and prevention* (Clinical Practice Guideline No. 3). Rockville, MD: Agency for Health Care Policy and Research.

This book is a summary of current research on methods for predicting and preventing pressure ulcers in adults. Although it was published about a decade ago, the recommendations have been revalidated in 2000. When followed, these guidelines assure best practice for pressure ulcer prevention for clients in any setting.

UNIT 8. FOCUSED PHYSICAL ASSESSMENT

8-1.   School-age Child Assessment

8-2.   Adult Assessment

8-1. SCHOOL-AGE ASSESSMENT

Learning Objectives

The learner is expected to:

1. Perform and document an appropriate focused physical assessment in an emergency situation.

2. Plan interventions for a life-threatening situation experienced by a child.

3. Plan and implement an interview of a parent whose child is suspected of being abused.

Critical Thinking Skill Practice and Validation

- Interpretation

- Explanation

- Inference

- Self-regulation

Critical Thinking Activity 8-1-1

You are a nurse for an elementary school. Today it is your turn to help monitor the students during recess on the playground. While playing, one of the first graders has a major seizure and falls off the swings. The other children run to tell you about this incident while a teacher calls 911 on her cell phone.

a.   When you see the child, what physical assessment should you perform first and why?

b.   Demonstrate a focused physical assessment of the child and document your findings below. Have another student, or your instructor, check your note for feedback.

c.   What initial interventions are appropriate for the child while waiting for the emergency personnel?

Critical Thinking Activity 8-1-2

When the emergency personnel arrive for the client described in Critical Thinking Activity 8-1-1, you accompany the child to the hospital because her mother has not yet been located. The child is now alert, but disoriented. After initial assessment in the Emergency Department, the nurse asks you if you have noticed the old and new bruising on the child's trunk and thighs. The mother of the child then runs into the ED demanding to see her "baby."

a.   How should the ED nurse conduct an interview of the mother? Pretend that your instructor or another student is the mother of this child and conduct the interview.

b.   What are the requirements for reporting suspected child abuse?

c.   What are possible explanations for the child's seizure?

Learning Objectives

The learner is expected to:

1. Perform a focused physical assessment on an older adult.

2. Perform a focused physical assessment on a middle-aged adult.

3. Perform a focused physical assessment on a young adult.

4. Document focused physical assessment findings.

5. Plan health teaching for a client with complex biopsychosocial problems.

Critical Thinking Skill Practice and Validation

- Explanation

- Analysis

- Evaluation

- Inference

- Self-regulation

Critical Thinking Activity 8-2-1

An older woman is admitted to the hospital from the nursing home with a diagnosis of urinary tract infection (UTI), sepsis, and dehydration. Her VS are 101^8-104-26, 154/92. Her pulse is weak and thready. A peripheral IV infusion of D5/0.45NS was started in the ED to run at 125 mL/h. The client is alert and oriented to person only. Her admission height and weight are 5'3" and 140 lbs. The client's health history includes a previous ischemic stroke, left below-the-knee amputation (BKA), colon cancer, and Nissen fundoplication for a large hiatal hernia.

a.   What priority assessments should you perform at this time and why?

b.   What abnormal laboratory results would you expect the client to have on admission and why? What urinary output would you expect?

c.   How will you determine when she is no longer dehydrated? How will you know if she receives too much fluid?

Critical Thinking Activity 8-2-2

A middle-aged man is admitted from home to the medical unit with multiple health problems, including cellulitis and gangrene of his right foot, peripheral vascular disease, obesity, coronary artery disease, osteoarthritis in both knees, history of lung cancer (right lung has been removed), and peptic ulcer disease. His wife left him last year because he is an alcoholic and "has trouble holding down a job." He lives alone, but says that a lady comes in every other week to clean and "do a little cooking." The client has no health insurance at this time because he is working part-time. He has no family in the area and few friends.

a.   What priority assessments should you perform at this time? Perform these assessments and document your findings. Have another student, or your instructor, check your note for feedback.

b.   What health teaching does this client need? What desired outcomes are realistic for him at this time? (Use the NOC system as a guide, if you are familiar with it.)

Critical Thinking Activity 8-2-3

A young woman driving a car is hit on the driver's side by a truck that ran the stoplight. You witness the accident and are the first responder at the scene. The woman is dazed and moaning in pain when you arrive. She tells you that her left arm hurts.

a.   What is the first assessment you should perform? Perform this assessment now. What other assessments will you perform?

b.   When you check her left arm, you observe that it is out of alignment and already beginning to swell. You suspect that her humerus is fractured; she also has surrounding tissue trauma. Perform an extremity assessment on the affected arm and document your findings here. Have another student, or your instructor, check your note for feedback.

Clinical Nursing Skills

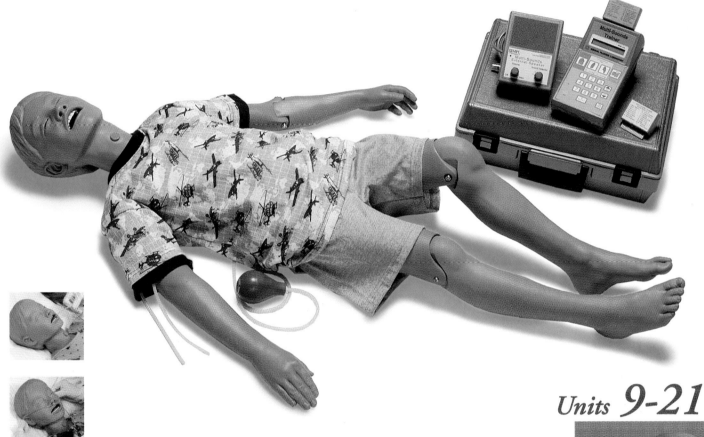

Units **9-21**

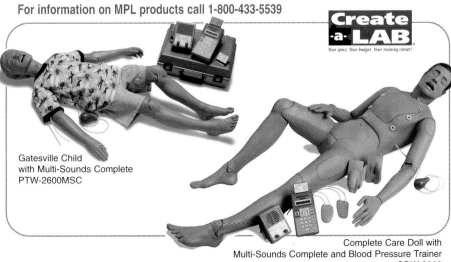

Gatesville Child
with Multi-Sounds Complete
PTW-2600MSC

Complete Care Doll with
Multi-Sounds Complete and Blood Pressure Trainer
GDW-3000

Clinical Nursing Skills

UNIT 9. INFECTION CONTROL

9-1.   Standard Precautions

9-2.   Isolation Precautions

Suggested Readings

9-1. STANDARD PRECAUTIONS

Learning Objectives

The learner is expected to:

1.   Identify protective measures that are included in Standard Precautions.

2.   Plan for staff education when needed to ensure compliance with Standard Precautions.

Critical Thinking Skill Practice and Validation

- Explanation

- Inference

- Analysis

Critical Thinking Activity 9-1-1

An adult client is admitted to the hospital with a severe exacerbation of her Crohn's disease. She reports having 15-20 diarrheal stools per day. She is receiving IV therapy and has a Foley catheter in place for strict intake and output measurements.

a.   You assign her basic care to a patient care tech who asks you if the client should be placed on special isolation precautions due to her diarrheal stools. How should you respond? What is the rationale for your response? *

b.   Should this client be placed in a private room. Why or why not? *

*These activities and questions are also appropriate for unlicensed personnel, such as nursing and medical assistants, and patient care technicians.

Critical Thinking Activity 9-1-2

While working in a nursing home this evening, you notice that a certified nursing assistant is walking down the hall with gloves on. She goes into a resident's room to take the resident off of the bedpan, then returns to the hall to pull a clean draw sheet from the linen cart. She continues to wear the same pair of gloves.

a. Is the nursing assistant following Standard Precautions? Why or why not? What should you say to the nursing assistant? Pretend a fellow student or your instructor is the nursing assistant and role play this situation. *

b. Demonstrate how the nursing assistant should have provided resident care using Standard Precautions.

*These activities and questions are appropriate for unlicensed personnel, including nursing and medical assistants, and patient care technicians.

Critical Thinking Activity 9-1-3

You are being oriented as a new graduate by an experienced nurse preceptor, who is showing you today how to start an IV. When you observe her technique, you note that she is having difficulty finding an appropriate vein in the client's forearm. You also observe that the nurse has long, acrylic nails that are well-manicured. The preceptor tears a hole in the end of her forefinger glove to help her palpate the vein. She tells you that she learned how to start IVs before gloves were mandatory, and she sometimes has problems feeling the vein with gloves on. She says she is not worried about blood-borne diseases because this is a small rural hospital and she knows almost everyone who is admitted.

a.   Did this preceptor follow Standard Precautions? Why or why not?

b.   As a new graduate, should you respond to the nurse's technique? Why or why not? Role play with another student or your instructor to demonstrate how you would handle this situation.

c.   Should nurses providing direct care for clients be allowed to have acrylic or sculptured nails? Why or why not?

9-2. ISOLATION PRECAUTIONS

Learning Objectives

The learner is expected to:

1. Determine what type of isolation precautions and barriers are needed for selected client situations.

2. Define common terms associated with infection control.

Critical Thinking Skill Practice and Validation

- Interpretation

- Analysis

- Inference

- Explanation

Critical Thinking Activity 9-2-1

A young college student is admitted to your unit with a probable diagnosis of *Haemophilus influenzae* type B meningitis. Several students from his school have been diagnosed with this disease.

a.   What isolation precautions will the client require based on his probable diagnosis and why? What infection control measures will the staff need to use to follow these precautions? *

b.   Will the client require a private room during his hospital stay? Why or why not?

c.   If he is scheduled to leave his room for a diagnostic test, what precautions are necessary?

*These activities and questions are also appropriate for unlicensed personnel, such as nursing and medical assistants, and patient care technicians.

Critical Thinking Activity 9-2-2

An older adult in a nursing home is diagnosed with methicillin-resistant *Staphylococcus aureus* (MRSA), which has colonized in both his urine and sacral pressure ulcer. The resident is currently in a semi-private room. As the charge nurse, you are responsible for educating the staff about the precautions that this resident will require.

a.   What isolation precautions will be necessary for this resident and why? What protective barriers will the staff need to use? *

b.   Will the resident need to be moved to a private room? Why or why not? *

*These activities and questions are also appropriate for unlicensed personnel, such as nursing and medical assistants, and patient care technicians.

143

Review of Terms 9-2-3

Match the term in the left column with its definition from the right column.

___1. Pathogen

A. Antigen-antibody response

___2. Antibiotic

B. Barrier used for airborne isolation precautions

___3. Handwashing

C. A disease-producing microorganism

___4. Barrier

D. The most important method for preventing infection

___5. Protective isolation

E. Medication that kills bacteria

___6. Particulate filter mask

F. Any measure to prevent spread of infection

___7. Septicemia

G. A protein that destroys antigens in the body

___8. Immunization

H. Use of barriers for an immuno-compromised client

___9. Humoral immunity

I. Infection in the blood

__10. Antibody

J. Medication that activates an immune response before exposure to the disease antigen

SUGGESTED READINGS

Hanchett, M. (1998). Implementing standard precautions in home care. *Home Care Management, 2*(2), pp. 16-20.

Many clients with infections are cared for at home. Measures need to be implemented to protect the other members of the household, as well as direct caregivers. The author recommends ways that families and other caregivers can be taught how to prevent the spread of infection, including frequent and proper handwashing techniques.

Sarver-Steffensen, J.A. (1999). When MRSA reaches into long-term care. *RN, 62*(3), pp. 39-41.

This article describes the growing incidence of multiply-resistant microorganisms among the nursing home population. Methicillin-resistant *S. aureus* is one of the most common problems and is quickly transmitted among residents unless careful isolation precautions are used.

Steed, C.J. (1999). Common infections in the hospital: The nurse's role in prevention. *Nursing Clinics of North America, 34*(2), pp. 443-461.

Nurses and assistive nursing personnel have a vital role in preventing the spread of infection among their clients. Proper and frequent handwashing, as well as meticulous adherence to Standard Precautions for all clients is essential. If infections are suspected that require airborne, droplet, or contact isolation precautions, nurses should implement these barriers immediately.

UNIT 10. WOUND CARE

10-1. Pressure Ulcer Care

10-2. Incision Care

Suggested Readings

10-1. PRESSURE ULCER CARE

Learning Objectives

The learner is expected to:

1. Apply selected clean dressings to pressure ulcers.

2. Explain the purpose of selected dressings.

3. Plan health teaching for caregivers providing wound care.

4. Analyze wound assessment data to determine the appropriate interventions.

5. Determine which wound dressing changes may be **delegated** to unlicensed assistive personnel.

Critical Thinking Skill Practice and Validation

- Analysis

- Explanation

- Inference

- Self-regulation

Critical Thinking Activity 10-1-1

You are assigned to care for a client at home who has a large draining Stage IV pressure ulcer and a smaller Stage II ulcer on his sacrum. Although the large ulcer is beginning to granulate, the client's wife has been applying wet-to-dry dressings twice a day to both ulcers as instructed two weeks ago by her husband's physician. Upon assessment of his wound, you note copious tan drainage and slough over 50% of the wound bed of the Stage IV ulcer. The tissue around the wound is reddened and hot. You decide to use an alginate dressing instead of the wet-to-dry dressing, and prepare to teach the wife how to apply the new dressing. You suggest a hydrocolloid dressing (Duoderm®) for the smaller lesion.

a.   Why are wet-to-dry dressings the least preferred treatments for these pressure ulcers? What is the advantage of this treatment?

b.   What is the primary purpose for an alginate dressing? Demonstrate how to apply the alginate dressing for this client's wound.

c.   What is the purpose of the Duoderm® dressing? Demonstrate how to apply this dressing. What instructions about this dressing should you provide for his wife?

d.   What action should you take related to the hot, reddened tissue that
       surrounds the larger pressure ulcer? Why?

Critical Thinking Activity 10-1-2

A middle-aged adult is admitted to your skilled nursing facility with Type II diabetes mellitus, h/o GI bleeding, hypokalemia (decreased serum potassium), and partial blindness. He also has a history of alcoholism. When performing his admission assessment, you note that he has a large gangrenous toe and a heel ulcer. The physician's order for skin care states, "Ulcer care per protocol."

a.   Assess his ulcer and document your findings below. Have another student, or your instructor, check your note for feedback.

b.   Apply appropriate gauze dressing to the heel ulcer using clean technique.

c.   Should this dressing be **delegated** to an unlicensed nursing staff member? Why or why not?

10-2. INCISION CARE

Learning Objectives

The learner is expected to:

1. Perform a wound irrigation using sterile technique.

2. Perform a dressing change using sterile technique.

3. Determine which wound dressing changes may be **delegated** to unlicensed assistive personnel.

4. Provide health teaching about incision care to a family caregiver.

Critical Thinking Skill Practice and Validation

- Analysis

- Explanation

- Inference

- Self-regulation

Critical Thinking Activity 10-2-1

You are assigned to a client in the hospital who has a clean, but gaping abdominal wound. The physician ordered a saline irrigation QD and packing with damp saline gauze to be covered by an abdominal pad and secured with Montgomery straps. The treatment is scheduled for 10:00 this morning.

a.   Should this dressing change be **delegated** to unlicensed assistive personnel? Why or why not?

b.   Should this dressing be applied using sterile technique? Why or why not?

c.   At 10AM the patient care tech reports that she has not yet had time to help the client with her bath. What should you do at this time?

d.   Perform the wound irrigation and dressing change. Also change the Montgomery straps and gauze ties.

Critical Thinking Activity 10-2-2

A surgeon is changing the initial postoperative dressing on a client who had abdominal surgery for colon cancer. The client has staples and a penrose drain in place. The client's wife asks the physician if she will need to learn how to change the client's dressing. He reassures her that the dressing and drain will be removed by discharge from the hospital, but that a small dry gauze may be needed over the drain site at home.

a.   The next day you need to change his dressing. Perform this procedure and document your assessment and treatment. Have another student, or your instructor, check your note for feedback.

b.   Before the client is discharged, the surgeon writes an order to "remove half of the staples." Perform this procedure.

c.   Pretend that a fellow student or your instructor is the client's wife. Provide health teaching about incision and drain site care at home.

Fowler, E., et al. (1999). Wound care for persons with diabetes. *Home Healthcare Nurse, 17*(7), pp. 437-444.

Clients with diabetes often have acute and chronic wounds, especially on the lower extremities. This article discussed wound assessment and management principles, including cleansing, debridement, and the use of moisture retentive dressings. Infection control is also an important intervention as part of wound care for the diabetic.

Hess, C.T. (2000). When to use alginate dressings. *Nursing2000, 30*(2), pp. 26.

This brief article explains the use of absorbent alginate dressings for wounds that are draining, most often Stage III and Stage IV pressure ulcers. These dressings remove necrotic tissue and fluid to allow for healing. Several types are available for use.

Krasner, D.L. & Sibbald, R.G. (1999). Nursing management of chronic wounds: Best practices across the continuum of care. *Nursing Clinics of North America, 34*(4), pp. 933-953.

Nurses care for clients with chronic, nonhealing wounds in a variety of health care settings. This article discussed best practices based on scientific evidence for management, including cleansing, irrigation, debridement, infection control, and topical treatment.

Senecal, S.J. (1999). Pain management of wound care. *Nursing Clinics of North America, 34*(4), pp. 847-860.

Assessing and managing pain is an important component for comprehensive wound care. Drug therapy and nonpharmacologic measures should be employed to ensure pain control during wound care and dressing changes.

UNIT 11. OXYGENATION SKILLS

11-1. Oxygen Administration / Pulse Oximetry

11-2. Oral and Nasotracheal Suctioning

11-3. Tracheostomy Care and Suctioning

11-4. Chest Physiotherapy / Incentive Spirometry

11-5. Chest Drainage Systems

Suggested Readings

Learning Objectives

The learner is expected to:

1. Explain the use of and precautions related to oxygen administration.

2. Explain the purpose of the oxygen analyzer.

3. Administer and monitor oxygen therapy.

4. Interpret pulse oximetry results.

5. Evaluate the effectiveness of oxygen therapy.

Critical Thinking Skill Practice and Validation

- Interpretation

- Explanation

- Inference

- Analysis

- Evaluation

Critical Thinking Activity 11-1-1

A 15-month old child with a severe respiratory infection is admitted to the pediatric unit. The physician ordered an oxygen tent at 40% oxygen concentration. The child's mother seems very anxious and asks you many questions. In collaboration with the respiratory therapist (RT), you assess the infant and set up the oxygen therapy.

a. The child's mother asks if she can bring some of the child's toys in for her daughter to play with. What advice should you give her?

b. The RT uses an oxygen analyzer as part of the monitoring process. What does this device measure and why is it an important part of the child's oxygen therapy?

c. The mother asks you later in the day why her daughter's pajamas feel damp. What explanation should you give her and what should you do at this time?

d.   If available, set up an oxygen tent.

e.   Why might the mother be anxious? What interventions could you use to allay her anxiety?

Critical Thinking Activity 11-1-2

An older adult is admitted to your medical unit from home with a diagnosis of pneumonia. His daughter tells you that he is usually alert, oriented and independent with his care, but today he has become lethargic and disoriented. She states that he seems very restless and "picks at" his bedcovers. His vital signs are 101-104-38, 162/94. When you check his pulse oximetry reading, it is 88%.

a.   Why do you think the client is lethargic and restless?

b.   The physician orders O_2 via NC at 4L/min. Implement this order now. Explain to the daughter (fellow student or instructor) the precautions that are needed with oxygen administration.

c.   After two hours of O_2 therapy, you check the client's "pulse ox" again. What should happen to the SaO_2 level? What is the difference between an SaO_2 and PaO_2 measurement? What other client outcomes should you expect?

d. What factors can affect the accuracy of a pulse oximetry measurement?

e. If the client had a history of pulmonary emphysema and CO_2 retention, would the oxygen order for 4L/min be appropriate? Why or why not?

11-2. ORAL AND NASOTRACHEAL SUCTIONING

Learning Objectives

The learner is expected to:

1. Determine if oral or nasotracheal suctioning should be **delegated** to unlicensed nursing personnel.

2. Provide health teaching related to suctioning for caregivers.

3. Perform nasotracheal suctioning on an adult and explain rationales for each step.

4. Evaluate the effectiveness of suctioning.

Critical Thinking Skill Practice and Validation

- Explanation

- Evaluation

- Inference

Critical Thinking Activity 11-2-1

You are a home care nurse visiting an older adult in her home as part of a hospice program. The client has had several surgeries, radiation and chemotherapy for oral cancer. As a result, she is unable to control her oral secretions and requires frequent oropharyngeal suctioning with a Yankauer catheter. You are here today to teach the daughter how to perform the suctioning procedure.

a.   Does this suctioning procedure require sterile technique? Why or why not?

b.   Pretend a fellow student or your instructor is the client's daughter and teach her how to suction the client.

c.   Is oropharyngeal suctioning a procedure that you could **delegate** to the home health aide? Why or why not?

Critical Thinking Activity 11-2-2

You are a nurse in a subacute care unit and are assigned today to care for a young adult who sustained a severe traumatic brain injury (TBI). He has been unconscious for several weeks and requires frequent nasotracheal suctioning of thick tenacious secretions to prevent aspiration.

a.   Should you **delegate** this procedure to an unlicensed nursing staff member? Why or why not?

b.   What physical assessment is needed before and after the client is suctioned?

c.   Demonstrate nasotracheal suctioning on this client. Be sure to explain the rationale for each step.

d.   What outcomes do you expect for the client as a result of suctioning and how will you know if they have been met?

11-3. TRACHEOSTOMY CARE AND SUCTIONING

Learning Objectives

The learner is expected to:

1. Perform tracheostomy care and suctioning and explain rationales for each step.

2. Perform appropriate physical assessment related to tracheostomy care and suctioning.

3. Document tracheostomy care and related physical assessment.

Critical Thinking Skill Practice and Validation

- Explanation

- Inference

- Self-regulation

Critical Thinking Activity 11-3-1

You are caring for a middle-aged man who had a partial laryngectomy and radical neck dissection for epiglottal cancer yesterday. He requires frequent tracheostomy suctioning and care. He is receiving morphine via a PCA pump for pain control and oxygen via a tracheostomy mask. When you explain the suctioning procedure to him, you discover that English is his second language. He uses paper and pen to communicate with you.

a.   What options do you have in the hospital setting to ensure that the client understands your health teaching and explanations?

b.   How will you determine when his tracheostomy needs to be suctioned?

c.   The physician ordered hyperoxygenation with a resuscitator bag during suctioning. Perform the tracheostomy suctioning and explain the rationales for each step. Will you need assistance with this procedure? Why or why not?

d. Another nurse tells you that she inserts a few milliliters of saline into a tracheostomy to loosen secretions before suctioning. Is this procedure considered best practice? Why or why not?

Critical Thinking Activity 11-3-2

After suctioning the client described in Critical Thinking Activity 11-3-1, you decide to perform tracheostomy care. The client's trach tube has a reusable inner cannula, and the ties are soiled with mucous secretions.

a.   Perform tracheostomy care and explain/write the rationales for each step.

b.   What precautions should you take during this procedure to prevent tracheostomy dislodgement?

c.   What emergency equipment should be present at the bedside for the client who has a new tracheostomy?

d.   Write a note to describe your physical assessment and tracheostomy care for this client. Have another student, or your instructor, check your note for feedback.

Learning Objectives

The learner is expected to:

1. Perform chest physiotherapy (PT), including percussion, vibration. and postural drainage, and document the procedure.

2. Identify contraindications and precautions associated with chest PT.

3. Teach an adult client how to use an incentive spirometer (IS) and perform deep breathing and coughing (DBC) exercises.

4. Explain the purpose of deep breathing and coughing exercises. and the use of the incentive spirometer for a postoperative client.

Critical Thinking Skill Practice and Validation

-   Explanation

-   Analysis

-   Inference

-   Self-regulation

Critical Thinking Activity 11-4-1

You are a nurse in a very small rural hospital. A middle-aged adult is admitted to the unit with bilateral lower lobe pneumonia and chronic bronchitis. He has been a smoker for 45 years, smoking 3 packs of unfiltered cigarettes per day. Although treated with oral antibiotics at home, his pneumonia has not resolved and he has become increasingly weak. The physician orders IV antibiotics, oxygen therapy, and chest physiotherapy (PT) twice a day.

a.   For how many pack-years has this client smoked?

b.   You prepare to do chest PT as ordered. (There is no respiratory therapist in your hospital.) When is the best time to perform this treatment? Demonstrate how to perform percussion, vibration, and postural drainage for this client. Remember to perform a physical assessment before and after the procedure.

c.   Document the procedure including physical assessment findings in the space below. Have another student, or your instructor, check your note for feedback.

Critical Thinking Activity 11-4-2

An older adult had a partial gastrectomy (stomach removal) yesterday and has been having difficulty using the incentive spirometer and performing deep breathing and coughing exercises. She tells you that her surgical area hurts worse when she tries the spirometer because it makes her cough. She is receiving continuous morphine via a PCA pump with a bolus option to control pain. The client tells you that she tries to "stay very still" so that the pain doesn't get too bad. Today, you also need to get her out of bed into a chair, which she refuses.

a.   What action should you take at this time so that the client can comply with the respiratory interventions that she needs postoperatively?

b.   What is the primary purpose for aggressive postoperative respiratory therapies?

c.   Teach the client how to deep breathe and cough (DBC) so that she can support her incisional area. Use another student or your instructor for this activity.

d.   Teach the client how to use the incentive spirometer (IS). Use another student or your instructor for this activity.

e.   Why is it essential that this client get out of bed today?

11- 5. CHEST DRAINAGE SYSTEMS

Learning Objectives

The learner is expected to:

1.   Compare and contrast commonly used chest drainage systems.

2.   Explain the nursing interventions that are required when caring for a client with a chest drainage system.

3.   Determine legal implications for not following best practice interventions based on research evidence.

4.   Define common terms related to chest drainage systems and other respiratory care.

Critical Thinking Skill Practice and Validation

- Analysis

- Inference

- Explanation

Critical Thinking Activity 11-5-1

As part of your client assignment today on the cardiothoracic unit, you have two clients who have chest drainage systems. One client has a single chest tube that was inserted yesterday for a left pneumothorax. The chest tube is connected to a one-bottle drainage system. The other client has two chest tubes that are connected to a disposable water-seal suction system. This client had part of his right lung removed for lung cancer through a thoracotomy two days ago.

a.   Why do these two clients have different chest drainage systems?

b.   Which system is connected to wall suction?

c.   What nursing care is necessary to manage clients who have chest drainage systems and why?

Critical Thinking Activity 11-5-2

While reading the previous shift nurse's notes regarding the client with the water-seal suction system in Critical Thinking Activity 11-5-1, you note where she "milked and stripped" the chest tubes. When you ask your manager about this procedure, she tells you that nurses need a physician's order to do the procedure. Neither client has an order on the chart.

a.   What is "milking and stripping," and why is it no longer routinely considered as part of best practice for chest tube care?

b.   What should you do in this situation?

c.   What are the legal issues involved in this situation?

Review of Terms 11-5-3

Match the term in the left column with its definition from the right column.

___1. Oxygen flowmeter

A. Surgical opening into the chest

___2. Humidification

B. Insertion of an artificial airway

___3. Pneumothorax

C. Alveolar collapse of the lung

___4. Venturi mask

D. A device used to keep a tracheostomy open if needed

___5. Atelectasis

E. A device that distributes oxygen and medication into the lungs

___6. Nebulizer

F. Adding water to the air

___7. Hemothorax

G. Air in the pleural space

___8. Intubation

H. An O_2 device that ensures precise O_2 concentrations

___9. Thoracotomy

I. Blood in the pleural space

__10. Obturator

J. A device that controls the amount of oxygen delivered in liters

Carroll, P. (2000). Exploring chest drain options. *RN, 63*(10), pp. 50-54.

A variety of chest drainage systems are now available for client problems. This article describes how these systems work and what nursing care and monitoring is necessary. Complications of chest tubes and drainage systems are also discussed.

Fox, V., et al. (1999). Patients' experiences of having an underwater seal chest drain. *Journal of Clinical Nursing, 8*(6), 684-692.

The authors describe a small study to determine client preparation and pain management when they have one or more chest tubes. Findings included lack of preparation preoperatively for chest tube insertion and lack of adequate pain management during insertion, maintenance, and removal of the tubes. Clients reported the pain as moderate to severe intensity, and described it as typical of somatic/visceral pain. This study was replicated two years later using a larger sample, and the findings were similar.

McConnell, E.A. (2000). Suctioning a tracheostomy tube. *Nursing2000, 30*(1), pp. 80.

This brief article highlights the steps for properly suctioning a tracheostomy using sterile technique. Photos accompany the text to clearly illustrate the correct technique.

UNIT 12. CARDIOVASCULAR SKILLS

12-1. Antiembolism Stockings / Sequential Compression Devices

12-2. Central Venous Pressure

Suggested Readings

12-1. ANTIEMBOLISM STOCKINGS / SEQUENTIAL COMPRESSION DEVICES

Learning Objectives

The learner is expected to:

1. Apply antiembolism stockings (AES) and sequential compression devices (SCDs) correctly.

2. Determine if AES and SCD application can be **delegated** to unlicensed nursing staff members.

3. Explain the physical assessment and monitoring required for the client wearing AES and/or SCDs.

Critical Thinking Skill Practice and Validation

- Explanation

- Analysis

- Inference

Critical Thinking Activity 12-1-1

A nursing assistant reports to you that one of her clients is complaining that her thighs hurt from wearing thigh-high elastic stockings. When you check the client, you find that she has pushed both stockings down to her knees and there is a deep U-shaped indentation in the skin of both thighs. You suspect that the stockings have been placed on her legs wrong side out.

a.　What is the purpose of thigh-high antiembolism stockings (AES)? Why are they preferred over knee-high stockings? *

b.　Determine the correct size for this client's antiembolism stockings and apply them correctly. Is this a skill that can be **delegated** to an unlicensed nursing staff member? Why or why not?

c.　What nursing care is required for the client who should wear AES? How often should they be removed?

*These activities and questions are appropriate for unlicensed personnel, such as nursing and medical assistants, and patient care technicians.

Critical Thinking Activity 12-1-2

You are caring for a client who has returned from the OR following a total hip replacement. The physician order requires application of thigh-high sequential compression devices (SCDs) over antiembolism stockings. The client also has an abduction pillow in place.

a.   What is the purpose of SCDs? Can the application of SCDs be **delegated** to unlicensed nursing personnel? Why or why not? *

b.   What precautions should be considered in applying and maintaining these devices? *

c.   What physical assessment is required for a client using SCDs?

*These activities and questions are also appropriate for unlicensed personnel, such as nursing assistants and patient care technicians.

12-2. CENTRAL VENOUS PRESSURE

Learning Objectives

The learner is expected to:

1. Explain the purpose of central venous pressure (CVP) measurement as part of hemodynamic monitoring.

2. Take an accurate CVP measurement.

3. Interpret findings from CVP measurements and take appropriate action, if needed.

Critical Thinking Skill Practice and Validation

- Interpretation

- Explanation

- Inference

Critical Thinking Activity 12-2-1

A client is admitted to the medical unit from critical care with a central venous pressure (CVP) manometer. His CVP readings have ranged between 6 and 9 for the past 24 hours. You are assigned to care for the client today.

a.   What is the purpose of monitoring central venous pressure?

b.   Demonstrate how to take a CVP measurement on this client.

c.   At what level should you hold the manometer to ensure an accurate reading? Why?

Critical Thinking Activity 12-2-2

Your first CVP measurement tonight on the client in Critical Thinking Activity 12-2-1 is 3 cm H_2O. You recheck it to make sure you measured correctly, and it remains a 3.

a.   What is the significance of this change in CVP measurement, if any?

b.   You notice during the process of measuring the client's CVP that the fluid level in the column fluctuates when the client breathes. Is this normal? Why or why not?

c.   What physical assessment should you perform at this time?

d.   What action should you take based on your measurement, if any? Why?

Ahrens, T. (1999). Hemodynamic monitoring. *Critical Care Nursing Clinics of North America, 11*(1), pp. 19-31.

This comprehensive article describes hemodynamic monitoring and its use in the critical care setting, especially the use of the pulmonary artery catheter. However, it is a complex and expensive technology and is associated with serious, though infrequent, complications. For that reason, it should be reserved for clients who need such invasive monitoring.

Toto, K.H. (1998). Fluid balance assessment: The total perspective. *Critical Care Nursing Clinics of North America, 10*(4), pp. 383-400.

The authors make the point that health care professionals have become too dependent on technology, such as hemodynamic monitoring, to determine a client's fluid balance status. Information gained from basic physical assessment skills and interpretation of common blood and urine laboratory values is equally, if not more, important as numbers derived by invasive monitoring techniques.

UNIT 13. URINARY ELIMINATION SKILLS

13-1. Urinary Catheters / Irrigation

13-2. Urine Specimens and Testing

Suggested Readings

Learning Objectives

The learner is expected to:

1. Catheterize a female client and document this intervention.

2. Catheterize a male client.

3. Explain the nursing care necessary when caring for a client with an indwelling urethral (Foley) catheter.

4. Explain the nursing care necessary when caring for a client with a suprapubic catheter.

5. Maintain a continuous bladder irrigation and interpret changes in urinary output.

6. Irrigate a Foley catheter.

7. Determine if catheter irrigation can be **delegated** to unlicensed assistive nursing personnel.

Critical Thinking Skill Practice and Validation

- Interpretation

- Explanation

- Analysis

- Self-regulation

Critical Thinking Activity 13-1-1

You are caring for an older adult who returned from the post anesthesia care unit (PACU) for a total knee replacement under epidural anesthesia 6 hours ago. She has not voided since surgery, but has received continuous IV fluids at 125 mL/hr. The client has been confused since admission and has pulled out her IV once since her surgery. When you call the surgeon, she gives you an order to "straight cath Q8h if not voided."

a.   Assess the client for urinary retention. What are possible reasons for the client not voiding?

b.   You prepare to catheterize the client. Do you think you will need assistance? Why or why not?

c.   Perform the urinary catheterization. Write a note below to document your actions and urinary output. Have another student, or your instructor, check your note for feedback.

Critical Thinking Activity 13-1-2

You have a physician's order for an indwelling urethral (Foley) catheter for one of your male clients. The client had a transurethral resection of the prostate gland (TURP) two years ago for benign prostatic hyperplasia (BPH). He is alert and oriented, and tells you he has had this procedure before.

a.   Demonstrate how to catheterize this client.

b.   If you had difficulty inserting the catheter, what action would you take?

c.   How should you secure a Foley catheter for a male client? Why is it different than for a female client?

d.   What precautions will you take when placing the urinary drainage bag?

Critical Thinking Activity 13-1-3

The client in Critical Thinking Activity 13-1-2 has another TURP. He returns from PACU with a continuous bladder irrigation (CBI) and a three-way Foley catheter. On admission to your unit, his urinary output is clear and slightly blood-tinged. You plan your care for the client.

a.   At the end of the shift, the client's intake is 360 mL PO and 900 mL bladder irrigant. His output in the drainage bag is 1900 mL. What is his total intake and actual urinary output?

b.   At the beginning of the next shift while rounding with you, the oncoming nurse notes that the client's urine has become cherry red, but not thickened. What action should you or the oncoming nurse take at this time?

c.   The physician orders intermittent irrigation with normal saline (NS) if the urinary catheter becomes blocked. Demonstrate how to perform this skill. Is this a skill that you would **delegate** to an unlicensed assistive nursing staff member? Why or why not?

Critical Thinking Activity 13-1-4

You admit a resident with a suprapubic (S/P) catheter to your nursing home from the hospital. He tells you that he is hoping that the catheter can be removed soon because it is uncomfortable. The physician has ordered a protocol that specifies clamping the S/P catheter every 3 hours and opening for 10 minutes while the resident is awake. At night, the catheter is connected to straight drainage.

a.   What is the purpose for the clamping protocol?

b.   What nursing care is needed for the client who has a S/P catheter?

c.   Change the dressing that is around the S/P catheter.

Critical Thinking Activity 13-1-5

An older man is admitted to your unit following a thrombotic stroke. He has left-sided weakness, urinary incontinence, and global aphasia. He has a history of Alzheimer's disease, and has been maintained prior to this admission at home in the care of his daughter. The daughter is very concerned that his skin will break down from urinary incontinence and requests that a Foley catheter be inserted.

a.   Do you think that a Foley catheter is the best option for this client? Why or why not? What other options could be tried first?

b.   Demonstrate at least two options for managing urinary incontinence for this client. What are the advantages and disadvantages of each option?

Learning Objectives

The learner is expected to:

1. Teach a client how to obtain a clean catch urine specimen.

2. Perform a dipstick test on a urine specimen and interpret findings.

3. Provide health teaching for a client with a urinary tract infection (UTI).

4. Explain the difference between asymptomatic bacteriuria and a UTI in the older adult.

Critical Thinking Skill Practice and Validation

- Interpretation

- Explanation

- Inference

- Analysis

Critical Thinking Activity 13-2-1

An adolescent girl comes to the clinic with complaints of burning on urination, frequency, and severe bladder pain. She states that she has been having this problem for several days, and it has worsened. When taking a history, she tells you that she has two children, is not married, and is sexually active. The client dropped out of high school last year, and works for a local fast food restaurant. Her mother watches the children while she is at work. The physician orders a clean catch urine specimen and a dipstick test for white blood cells.

a.   Obtain the necessary supplies and teach the client how to obtain a clean catch urine specimen. Be sure to use appropriate language for her educational level. Pretend another student or your instructor is the client.*

b.   What is the purpose of the dipstick testing for white blood cells (WBCs)? Perform this test if you have the supplies available.

c.   When you check the dipstick results, the client has 10+ WBCs. She also has a trace of blood in her urine. What might explain the blood in her urine?

d. The physician orders antibiotic therapy for her urinary tract infection (UTI). What health teaching should you provide for this client? What precautions might help prevent further UTIs in the future?

Critical Thinking Activity 13-2-2

The physician writes an order for a urine culture and sensitivity (C & S) for a nursing home resident with a long-term Foley catheter. The resident's urine is cloudy and contains mucous threads and sediment. Otherwise, he has no symptoms of a urinary tract infection.

a.   Would you question the physician's order for the C & S? Why or why not?

b.   What interventions should you implement that might improve the appearance of the resident's urine?

c.   Demonstrate how to collect a specimen from a closed urinary drainage system. Do you expect that the resident's urine will contain bacteria? Is this finding uncommon in nursing home residents who have long-term catheters?

d.   What is best practice regarding treating asymptomatic bacteriuria in older adults? Why?

Gray, M. (2000). Urinary retention. Management in the acute care setting, Part 2. *American Journal of Nursing, 100*(8), 36-43.

The author discusses the problem of urinary retention and common causes. Physical assessment to determine retention is described and options for management are outlined, including urinary catheterization. Risk factors, methods and equipment for this procedure are also discussed.

Newman, D.K. (1998). Managing indwelling urethral catheters. *Ostomy and Wound Management, 44*(12), pp. 26-28, 30, 32.

This article discusses the use of Foley catheters to manage urinary incontinence, neurogenic bladder and urinary retention. The author then reviews current strategies for providing good catheter management, as well as steps for retraining the client following catheter removal.

Smith, A.B. & Adams, L.L. (1998). Insertion of indwelling urethral catheters in infants and children: A survey of current practice. *Pediatric Nursing, 24*(3), pp. 229-234.

The authors studied current nursing practice standards for insertion of indwelling urinary catheters in infants and children using a sample of 46 hospitals to determine recommended guidelines. Findings revealed a wide variation in practice without scientific evidence or research base to support nursing policies. The authors concluded that standards must be consistent and based on knowledge of anatomical structure and the dimensions of available catheters.

UNIT 14. NUTRITION AND GASTROINTESTINAL SKILLS

14-1. NASOGASTRIC TUBES

Learning Objectives

The learner is expected to:

1. Explain the difference between a Salem sump and Levin nasogastric tube.

2. Insert a nasogastric (NG) tube.

3. Describe and document nursing care required for a client with an NG tube.

4. Irrigate a nasogastric tube and document findings.

5. Remove a nasogastric tube.

Critical Thinking Skill Practice and Validation

- Explanation

- Evaluation

- Inference

- Self-regulation

Critical Thinking Activity 14-1-1

A client is admitted to your unit with a diagnosis of intestinal obstruction. On assessment you find that she has a distended abdomen and recent nausea and vomiting. The physician orders an "Salem sump for decompression; irrigate QS with NS."

a.   What is the difference between a Salem sump and Levin nasogastric tube? When you insert the Salem sump tube, what setting will you use for the suction – low intermittent or low continuous – and why?

b.   Insert the tube into the client now. Be sure to secure the tube and connect it to suction.

c.   In what position should you keep the client while she has the tube in place and why? How would you know if the decompression was effective for this client?

d.   What nursing care and documentation is required for the client having an NG tube for decompression?

Critical Thinking Activity 14-1-2

The client in the Critical Thinking Activity 14-1-1 requires irrigation to maintain patency of her tube. When you prepare to irrigate the Salem sump, you find that the client is lying flat in bed and someone has tied the blue pigtail into a knot.

a.   What actions should you take now and why?

b.   Irrigate the tube with normal saline as ordered. How much solution should you use? Is this a sterile procedure? Why or why not? Document the results of the irrigation below, including intake and output. Have another student, or your instructor, check your note for feedback.

c.   Should you **delegate** NG tube irrigation to unlicensed assistive nursing personnel? Why or why not?

d.   Several days later, the physician orders the tube to be removed. Under what circumstances should nurses NOT remove a nasogastric tube?

e.   Remove the Salem sump tube.

f.   What physical assessment is needed before, during and after stomach decompression for this client?

Learning Objectives

The learner is expected to:

1. Initiate and maintain continuous enteral feedings via a nasoduodenal and gastrostomy tube.

2. Explain the difference between a Keofeed and Levin tube.

3. Describe the nursing assessment and interventions needed for the client receiving enteral feedings.

4. Check for proper placement of a feeding tube.

5. Intervene in potentially life-threatening situations for clients receiving enteral feedings and document appropriate actions.

6. Provide gastrostomy tube care.

Critical Thinking Skill Practice and Validation

- Explanation

- Inference

- Analysis

- Evaluation

- Self-regulation

Critical Thinking Activity 14-2-1

The nurse practitioner has ordered continuous tube feeding (Jevity®) at 50 ml/hr for a client who was transferred from acute care to your subacute unit. At the present time, the client has a Keofeed tube in place. An enteral feeding pump and open feeding bag system will be used for this client.

a.   What physical assessment is needed before you start the client's enteral feeding?

b.   How does a Keofeed tube differ from a Levin tube? What is the MOST reliable way to initially ensure proper placement of either tube? Demonstrate the method that you should use for checking tube placement at frequent intervals.

c.   Prepare the tube feeding for initiation. How much formula should you add to the bag at one time and why?

d.   Once you have started the continuous feeding, what monitoring and
        maintenance nursing activities are necessary?

e.   About 12 hours after the continuous tube feeding was started, the client
        becomes restless and experiences dyspnea. What should you do FIRST and
        why?

f.   Document your assessment and interventions that relate to the new situation
        in e. above. Have another student, or your instructor check, your note for
        feedback.

Critical Thinking Activity 14-2-2

One of your residents in a skilled nursing home unit has an order for continuous tube feeding via G-tube from 2PM to 6AM each day to allow for 8 hours of "down time." An additional 100 mL H_2O Q4h is ordered by the dietitian to meet her fluid requirements. You are working as the charge nurse on the 3-11 shift for the B unit.

a.   When you check the resident's G-tube site, you note that the skin is red and excoriated. The tube can be moved in and out of the opening for more than an inch and leakage occurs when it moves. What action should you take at this time?

b.   The nurse practitioner replaces the G-tube with a Foley catheter and orders Mycostatin powder for the yeast infection. Dress the G-tube site after applying the powder.

c.   At 10PM when you check for residual, you draw back 250 mL of tube feeding into the syringe. What does this mean? What should you do with the residual? Are there other actions that you should take? Document this situation and your interventions below. Have another student, or your instructor, check your note for feedback.

Bliss, D.Z. & Lehmann, S. (1999). Tube feeding: Administration tips. *RN, 62*(8), pp. 29-31.

The authors discuss the basics of tube feedings, including the types of tubes that can be used, when and how to start feedings, and common complications that result from either the feeding formula or the tube. Aspiration and diarrhea are two of the most common problems associated with enteral feeding.

Edwards, S.J. & Metheny, N.A. (2000). Measurement of gastric residual volume: State of the science. *MEDSURG Nursing, 9*(3), pp. 125-128.

This article reviews the issue of determining what constitutes excessive gastric residual volume in adult tube-fed clients. Only one study was found that indicated that 200 mL for a nasogastric tube and 100 mL for a gastrostomy tube should be considered as excessive.

Ellett, M.L. & Beckstrand, J. (1999). Examination of gavage tube placement in children. *Journal of the Society of Pediatric Nursing, 4*(2), 51-60.

The findings of this descriptive study of 39 hospitalized children found that feeding tube placement error occurred in 43.5% of tubes inserted during the observation period. Children who were comatose or semi-comatose, were inactive, had swallowing tubes, or had Argyle tubes were more likely to have placement errors.

Metheny, N.A., Smith, L., & Stewart, B.J. (2000). Development of a reliable and valid bedside test for improving prediction of feeding tube location. *Nursing Research, 49*(6), pp. 302-309.

The researchers studied the effectiveness of bilirubin teststrips in determining feeding tube placement in combination with pH testing of gastric contents. A pH greater than 5 and a bilirubin less than 5mg/dL successfully identified 100% of the cases in which the tube was placed in the respiratory tract. A pH of less than 5 and bilirubin less than 5 mg/mL successfully identified 98% of cases in which the tube was in the stomach. The authors concluded that bilirubin testing used in combination with pH testing improves the ability to determine nasoenteral tube placement.

UNIT 15. BOWEL ELIMINATION SKILLS

15-1. Enema Administration / Fecal Occult Blood Test (FOBT)

15-2. Colostomy / Ileostomy Care

Suggested Readings

Learning Objectives

The learner is expected to:

1. Interpret the significance of bowel elimination problems.

2. Give a large-volume enema to an older adult.

3. Perform a fecal occult blood test (FOBT).

4. Determine when enema administration or FOBT can be **delegated** to unlicensed nursing personnel and provide rationale for the decision.

5. Give a small-volume enema to a child and document results.

Critical Thinking Skill Practice and Validation

-   Interpretation

-   Analysis

-   Inference

-   Explanation

-   Self-regulation

Critical Thinking Activity 15-1-1

An older adult is admitted to the hospital with hyperglycemia and pneumonia. She has been receiving warfarin (Coumadin) for a total hip replacement that she had two weeks ago. The nursing assistant tells you that the client has not had a bowel movement (BM) for three days, but is not complaining of abdominal discomfort.

a.   What should your FIRST action be and why?

b.   You decide to make the physician aware of the client's condition. He orders "Dulcolax 2 tabs tonight; if no BM by tomorrow afternoon, give tap water enema X1." Demonstrate how to give a large-volume enema to this client.

c.   Because the client receives Coumadin, you decide to test her stool for occult blood using a Hemocult test. Demonstrate how to do this FOBT and record the results below. What will you do if the results are positive for blood?

d.   Should the enema administration or FOBT be **delegated** to your patient care technician? Why or why not?

Critical Thinking Activity 15-1-2

A 10-year old obese boy is brought to the Emergency Department (ED) by his mother with complaint of abdominal distention, anorexia and obstipation. He is very anxious and tearful. The child's mother tells you that he sometimes goes a week or more without having a BM, but this time it has been 10 days. His appetite was not affected until three days ago. She gave him laxatives for the past two nights, but they have not been successful.

a.   The ED physician examines the child and orders an oil retention enema followed by a regular Fleets enema. Why are two different enemas ordered and how are they different?

b.   Give either type of enema to this client. Be sure to provide emotional support to help allay his anxiety. In the space below, document this procedure and its results, as well as your physical assessment. Have another student, or your instructor, check your note for feedback.

c.   The ED techs are allowed to give enemas. Should you delegate either or both enemas to one of your techs to give the client? Why or why not?

15-2. COLOSTOMY / ILEOSTOMY CARE

Learning Objectives

The learner is expected to:

1. Explain and identify the difference between a healthy and unhealthy ostomy stoma.

2. Document appropriate assessments and actions for a client who has an unhealthy stoma.

3. Plan individualized care, including health teaching, for a client having an ostomy.

4. Explain the difference between a colostomy and ileostomy.

5. Identify expected outcomes for the client with an ileostomy.

Critical Thinking Skill Practice and Validation

- Explanation

- Analysis

- Inference

- Self-regulation

Critical Thinking Activity 15-2-1

You are a nurse working in a continuing care retirement community. One of your residents, who had surgery for colorectal cancer, calls you and asks if you would see her today. She is concerned about the appearance of her colostomy stoma.

a.   When you assess the resident, you note that the stoma is not healthy. Document your assessment below, including the actions you plan to take. Have another student, or your instructor, check your note for feedback.

b.   The resident tells you that she is very overwhelmed by the new colostomy. She is not sure if she will be able to manage it. She is also afraid that her husband won't want to help her with such a "dirty thing." How should you respond?

c.   Teach the client how to change her two-piece appliance system and how to maintain her ostomy. Pretend that another student or your instructor is the client.

d. The resident asks you if she will always need to wear an appliance. Her colostomy is located in her LLQ. What should you tell her?

e. What stool consistency is expected from this colostomy? Is she a possible candidate for irrigation? Why or why not?

Critical Thinking Activity 15-2-2

A young woman is told that she needs an ileostomy for her Crohn's disease. She has recently become engaged and cries when her surgeon presents the ileostomy as the best option to control her disease.

a.   As the office nurse, how might you respond to her at this time? Is her reaction unusual? Support your answer.

b.   The client later decides to have the surgery. She asks you what the difference is between a colostomy and ileostomy. What should you tell her? Will she need to wear an appliance continuously?

c.   What outcomes are expected for this client? What other members of the health care team will you as her nurse need to collaborate with to meet these outcomes?

Ball, E.M. (2000). Ostomy guide. Part two: A teaching guide for continent ileostomy. *RN, 63*(12), pp. 35-38.

A continent ileostomy is an alternative to the traditional ileostomy for which a bag is continuously worn for drainage collection. This option allows for control of the drainage by the client by creating a reservoir, which is drained intermittently. The author presents information that will assist the nurse in health teaching for a client with this type of ileostomy.

Moppett, S. (1999). Administration of an enema. *Nursing Times, 95*(22), pp. 1-2.

This article reviews methods and contraindications for enema administration. Nursing considerations and assessment are discussed as important components of the procedure. Types of enemas are also described.

O'Brien, B.K. (1999). Coming of age with an ostomy: Life with a stoma may be especially difficult for teens. *American Journal of Nursing, 99*(8), 71-76.

The author reviews the developmental tasks associated with adolescence to emphasize the difficulty that teens have when dealing with having an ostomy. At this time in their lives, they are forming intimate relationships and having an ostomy makes them feel unattractive. The article provides excellent tips when working with teens who have stomas.

UNIT 16. MOBILITY SKILLS

16-1. Crutch Walking

16-2. Traction and Casts

Suggested Readings

Learning Objectives

The learner is expected to:

1.   Demonstrate how to measure a client for crutches.

2.   Demonstrate how to teach a client how to use crutches, including ambulating on stairs, and document the health teaching.

3.   Determine appropriate crutch walking gaits for selected clients.

Critical Thinking Skills Practice and Validation

- Analysis

- Explanation

- Evaluation

- Self-regulation

Critical Thinking Activity 16-1-1

A young adult fell while skiing and comes to the walk-in clinic where you are a nurse. Medical evaluation indicates that she has a right knee injury, most likely a severe ligament tear. The client is given a set of adjustable crutches and instructed to avoid weight bearing on the right leg until seen by an orthopedic surgeon.

a.   Demonstrate how to measure the client properly for crutches. Use a fellow student or your instructor for this activity.

b.   What crutch-walking gait would be the best to ensure that she is nonweight bearing (NWB) on her right leg? Why?

c.   Pretend that a fellow student or instructor is the client and teach him/her how to use the gait in b. above.

Critical Thinking Activity 16-1-2

A middle-aged adult has a left total hip replacement (THR) and is allowed to partial weight bear (PWB). The physical therapist teaches him the three-point crutch-walking gait.

a.   On your rehabilitation unit, the client gets out of bed using crutches. You observe him to ensure that he is using the correct procedure. Have a fellow student, or your instructor, use the three-point gait and evaluate if he/she is using it correctly.

b.   The client tells you that he has three steps leading to both doors of his home. He is concerned about using crutches on steps. Teach him the procedure by demonstrating it and have him perform a return demonstration. (Use a fellow student, or instructor, for this activity.)

c.   Document your health teaching below. Have another student, or your instructor, check for feedback.

Learning Objectives

The learner is expected to:

1.   Explain the nursing responsibilities associated with care of the client with selected types of traction and casts.

2.   Explain the difference between external and internal fixation.

3.   Describe the care needed for clients who have a casted extremity.

4.   Document physical assessment findings for a client with an external fixation device.

5.   Interpret abnormal physical assessment findings for a client who is casted.

6.   Define common terms associated with traction and casts.

Critical Thinking Skill Practice and Validation

•   Explanation

•   Interpretation

•   Evaluation

•   Self-regulation

•   Analysis

Critical Thinking Activity 16-2-1

You are caring for a 20-month old child who suffered a fractured left femur in a car accident and is placed in Bryant's traction preoperatively. Last week when you worked on the adult surgical unit, you had a client with Buck's traction.

a.   What type of traction is Bryant's traction? How is it similar and how is it different from Buck's traction? What is the purpose of this type of traction?

b.   What nursing responsibilities do you have when caring for a client in any type of traction?

c.   What physical assessment should you perform while the child is in Bryant's traction?

Critical Thinking Activity 16-2-2

A young adult suffered a crushing lower leg injury and tibia-fibula fractures when his motorcycle fell on him two days ago. You are assigned to care for him today. On assessment you find that he is receiving morphine via a PCA pump and has his left leg elevated on two pillows to support the Hoffman external fixator that was applied to his injured extremity.

a. How is external fixation different from an internal fixation procedure? What is the purpose of the Hoffman device?

b. What nursing responsibilities do you have when caring for a client with an external fixator?

c. What physical assessment will you perform on this client? Perform the assessment and document your findings below. Have another student, or your instructor, check note for feedback.

Critical Thinking Activity 16-2-3

A middle-aged client fell on the ice when getting into her car. In the ED, the physician applies a synthetic forearm cast for a radial fracture.

a.   As the ED nurse, what health teaching should you provide for the client?

b.   What physical assessment is needed for a client who has an extremity cast?

c.   Several days later, the client returns to the ED with complaints of a burning sensation under her cast. What is a possible explanation for this finding?

d.   Document your physical assessment for the situation in c. above, including what action that the physician will most likely take. Have another student, or your instructor, check note for feedback.

Review of Terms 16-2-4

Match the term in the left column with its definition in the right column.

____1. Russell's traction

A. Soft tissue injury resulting from blunt trauma

____2. Stryker frame

B. Skeletal traction used for long-term immobilization of fractures

____3. Buck's traction

C. Skin traction for a small child with a femur fracture

____4. Continuous passive motion (CPM) machine

D. Special bed for clients with spinal cord injury (SCI)

____5. External fixation device

E. Device for immobilizing the cervical spine

____6. Contusion

F. Skin traction used for fractured hip

____7. Bryant's traction

G. A device connected to skeletal traction to keep femur aligned

____8. Pearson attachment

H. Device used to promote joint mobility, usually postoperatively

____9. Halo traction

I. Skeletal traction used for femoral shaft fractures

___10. Thomas splint

J. Metal frame with percutaneous pins to maintain bone alignment while soft tissue heals

Byrne, T. (1999). The set-up and care of a patient in Buck's traction. *Orthopaedic Nursing, 18*(2), pp. 79-83.

This excellent article discusses every aspect of working with a client with Buck's traction, from setting the traction up to ongoing care of the client. Physical assessment and implications for best practice are clearly described.

Church, V. (2000). Staying on guard for DVT and PE. *Nursing2000, 30*(2), pp. 35-42.

Although deep vein thrombosis and pulmonary embolus do not occur solely in clients with musculoskeletal injury or surgery, a very large percentage of these life-threatening problems are found in this client population. Therefore, this article carefully describes how to prevent, monitor, and detect these health thromboembolitic problems, as well as discusses typical management.

Turner, L.W. et al. (1999). Osteoporosis diagnosis and fracture. *Orthopaedic Nursing, 18*(5), pp. 21-27.

The authors identify osteoporosis as a growing problem as the geriatric population increases. Many older adults are not diagnosed until they experience a fracture. The article discusses how the problem should be diagnosed early and the consequences of this problem, including potentially life-threatening hip fractures.

UNIT 17. MEDICATION ADMINISTRATION SKILLS

17-1. Oral and Enteral Medications

17-2. Sublingual and Topical Medications

17-3. Eye and Ear Medications

17-4. Vaginal and Rectal Medications

17-1. ORAL AND ENTERAL MEDICATIONS

Learning Objectives

The learner is expected to:

1. Calculate pediatric dosing for liquid medications.

2. Provide health teaching related to pediatric medication dosing.

3. Calculate medication dosing for adults.

4. Provide health teaching for selected adult clients related to medication administration.

5. Demonstrate how to give oral medications and document procedure.

6. Demonstrate how to administer medications via a gastrostomy tube and document.

Critical Thinking Skill Practice and Validation

- Interpretation

- Analysis

- Explanation

- Self-regulation

Critical Thinking Activity 17-1-1

The pediatrician orders cefprozil (Cefzil) suspension for a 13-month old infant for a respiratory infection. The child weighs 18 pounds. The recommended dosage is 15 mg/kg Q12 h X 10 days. The suspension is available as 125 mg/5mL.

a. How much cefprozil should the client's mother give to the child? Show your work below. Have another student, or your instructor, check your work for feedback.

b. As the office nurse, what should you teach the child's mother about the drug, including its storage? Pretend that another student, or your instructor, is the mother and provide health teaching.

Critical Thinking Activity 17-1-2

A middle-aged client is started on captopril (Capoten, Novo-Captopril~) at 6.25 mg BID by the nurse practitioner in the medical clinic. The client calls you after having his prescription filled and asks about his medication.

a.   The client has captopril 12.5 mg tablets on hand. How much should he take to ensure that he gets the intended dosage? Show your work below.

b.   What type of anti-hypertensive is this medication? What health teaching should you provide for the client regarding this medication? Pretend that another student or your instructor is the client and provide the necessary health teaching.

Critical Thinking Activity 17-1-3

A client was discharged from the behavioral health unit with a diagnosis of acute depression and suicidal tendencies. On discharge, the client was prescribed to continue on venlataxine HCl (Effexor XR) 150 mg QD.

a.   The capsules that are available from the local pharmacy are 75 mg each. How many capsules should you tell the client to take? What does XR indicate? Show your work below.

b.   The client states that the capsules are too difficult for him to swallow. What options does the client have to get the intended drug dose?

c.   Provide health teaching for this client, including side effects of the medication. Pretend that another student or your instructor is the client and provide the teaching.

Critical Thinking Activity 17-1-4

You are preparing to give medications at 10AM via a gastrostomy tube (G-tube). The medication administration record (MAR) indicates the medications prescribed by the physician's assistant to be given at 10AM:

- Dilantin 200 mg QD to prevent seizures

- Morphine Liquid 20 mg Q4h for chronic malignant pain

- Lanoxin Elixer 0.125 mg QD for CHF

- Colace Syrup 100 mg QD

a.   When you check the Dilantin order, what problem do you note and what options do you have to resolve it?

b.   The available Morphine Liquid is 20mg/5mL. How much should you give? Show your work below.

c.   The available Lanoxin Elixer is 0.05 mg/mL. How much should you give?

d.   When you are preparing to give these medications, what position should you place the client in and why?

e.   Demonstrate the procedure for administering medications via a G-tube and document on the MAR. Have another student, or your instructor, check it.

f.   When you are giving tablets or capsules via an enteral feeding tube, which medications should not be crushed (tablets) or opened (capsules) and why?

Learning Objectives

The learner is expected to:

1. Identify the purpose of selected sublingual (SL) and topical medications.

2. Provide health teaching about selected SL and topical medications.

3. Document health teaching about selected SL and topical medications.

Critical Thinking Skill Practice and Validation

- Explanation

- Self-regulation

- Evaluation

Critical Thinking Activity 17-2-1

An older client tells you in the physician's office that she is not sure about the "little white pills in the brown bottle" that she is supposed to give her husband for chest pain. She further states that she plans to call 911 if he experiences pain. When you look at the bottle, you determine that it is nitroglycerin (NTG) gr 1 150 SL.

a.   What health teaching should you provide about NTG for her husband? Pretend that another student or your instructor is the client and provide appropriate teaching. Document your teaching below.

b.   The client's daughter tells you that her aunt takes NTG in a spray form. How is the spray administered?

Critical Thinking Activity 17-2-2

A new mother has a prescription for triamcinolone acetonide (Kenalog cream) QID for dermatitis on her hands. You are visiting her in the home for a mother-baby visit.

a.   What is missing from this order for the topical medication?

b.   What health teaching should you provide for her? Document this activity and have another student, or your instructor, check note for feedback. (Be sure to include how to apply the medication.)

Critical Thinking Activity 17-2-3

A client is planning to take a cruise and desires to use a patch to prevent "seasickness." The physician prescribes Transderm Scop 1.5 mg/2.5 cm^2.

a.   The physician tells the client that one patch will last for 72 hours. How many mg will the client receive each day? Show your work below.

b.   Provide health teaching for this client, including how to administer each patch.

17-3. EYE AND EAR MEDICATIONS

Learning Objectives

The learner is expected to:

1. Compare the use of ophthalmic ointments and drops.

2. Demonstrate how to apply ophthalmic ointment and drops.

3. Explain the expected effect of selected ophthalmic drops.

4. Provide health teaching for clients receiving ophthalmic drops.

5. Demonstrate how to apply ear drops.

Critical Thinking Skill Practice and Validation

- Explanation

- Analysis

- Self-regulation

- Evaluation

Critical Thinking Activity 17-3-1

The physician orders gentamicin sulfate (Garamycin) ointment 0.3% to be administered in the resident's right eye QN X 7 days for conjunctivitis. The resident is unable to apply the medication herself.

a.   Demonstrate how to apply this medication. What is the abbreviation for the right eye?

b.   What is the advantage of an ophthalmic ointment when compared to ophthalmic drops? What is the disadvantage of ophthalmic ointments?

Critical Thinking Activity 17-3-2

A client in the home has a new prescription for 2% pilocarpine (Pilostat) two gtts QID OS for glaucoma. The client's husband does not know how to give the medication properly.

a.   Provide health teaching and demonstrate how to administer the eye drops as ordered. Pretend that another student or your instructor is the client's husband and provide the teaching.

b.   What is this drug's classification? What effect should the medication have on the client's eyes?

Critical Thinking Activity 17-3-3

A physician prescribes Otocort drops (two gtts in the left ear) for a 3-year old who has otitis media. The child's grandmother is the child's guardian and asks you how to administer the medication.

a.   Demonstrate how to give the eardrops for a small child.

b.   What health teaching should you provide about this medication, including its purpose and side/adverse effects?

17- 4. VAGINAL AND RECTAL MEDICATIONS

Learning Objectives

The learner is expected to:

1.   Demonstrate how to administer selected vaginal and rectal medications.

2.   Provide health teaching related to vaginal and rectal medication administration.

3.   Identify the expected outcomes for selected vaginal or rectal medications.

4.   Define common terms associated with nonparenteral medications.

Critical Thinking Skill Practice and Validation

- Explanation

- Evaluation

- Self-regulation

Critical Thinking Activity 17-4-1

A female client has a vaginal yeast infection and is prescribed Monistat 3 200 mg HS X 3. She complains of itching and a thick, "cottage cheese-like" vaginal drainage. During her health history, she tells you that she is sexually active and has these infections often.

a.   What instructions should you provide about how to administer this medication?

b.   Why should the drug be given at night?

c.   What other health teaching should you provide for her regarding sexual health?

Critical Thinking Activity 17-4-2

A pediatric nurse practitioner prescribes Dulcolax suppository PR for a 6 year-old child. The mother is anxious about giving the medication.

a.   What outcome should you tell the mother to expect after giving the suppository and how long should it take to work?

b.   Demonstrate how to give the suppository as part of your health teaching for the child's mother.

Review of Terms 17-4-3

Match the term in the left column with its definition from the right column.

___1. Suspension   A. Any medication applied to the skin

___2. Miotic   B. Applied or instilled into the eye

___3. Elixer   C. Liquid medication containing alcohol

___4. Capsule   D. Pupil dilator

___5. Topical   E. Under the tongue

___6. Otic   F. Thick liquid medication that separates into liquid and solid

___7. Transdermal   G. Pupil constrictor

___8. Sublingual   H. Applied into the ear

___9. Mydriatic   I. Gelatin-encased oral medication

__10. Ophthalmic   J. Topical application that permits medication administration at a fixed rate

UNIT 18. MEDICATION ADMINISTRATION SKILLS (PARENTERAL)

18-1. SUBCUTANEOUS AND INTRADERMAL MEDICATIONS

Learning Objectives

The learner is expected to:

1. Interpret a sliding scale for insulin administration.

2. Demonstrate how to administer and document subcutaneous and intradermal injections.

3. Explain the appropriate use of insulin therapy.

4. Compare major types of insulin.

5. Analyze the effects of insulin therapy.

6. Compare enoxaparin (Lovenox) and heparin therapy.

7. Calculate drug dosing for an adult client.

Critical Thinking Skill Practice and Validation

- Interpretation

- Analysis

- Explanation

- Inference

- Evaluation

- Self-regulation

Critical Thinking Activity 18-1-1

The physician orders sliding scale insulin, and NPH insulin 22 units QAM and 10 units QHS for a client admitted to the hospital with uncontrolled diabetes mellitus. The sliding scale order reads as follows:

Give Humulin-R per sliding scale AC and HS—

>400	10 u
350-400	8 u
300-349	6 u
250-299	4 u
200-249	3 u

a.   When should you assess the client's finger stick blood sugar (FSBS)? Take the client's FSBS if the equipment is available.

b.   What type of insulin is Humulin-R? Why is it the best choice for a sliding scale? What is its onset, peak action and duration of action?

c.   Give the client his insulin based on a FSBS of 322 at 11:30 AM. Document your medication administration on the appropriate medical records. How did you decide where to give the injection?

d.   Why is the client receiving two types of insulin?

e.   When is this client most at risk for hypoglycemia and why?

Critical Thinking Activity 18-1-2

You are caring for a postoperative client who has had a total hip replacement. The surgeon orders "Enoxaparin (Lovenox) 40 mg SC Q12 hrs. Begin warfarin (Coumadin) on POD #3."

a.   What is enoxaparin and how is it different from heparin?

b.   Demonstrate how to give the client this medication and document your action, including site selection. (The vial reads 40 mg/0.4mL.)

c.   What laboratory tests, if any, should you monitor for this client and why?

d.   What side/adverse effects should you monitor for and why?

e.   What additional concern should you have if the client had epidural anesthesia and/or analgesia?

f.   Why did the surgeon order warfarin while the client is receiving Lovenox SC?

Critical Thinking Activity 18-1-3

You are visiting a client at home on continuous ambulatory peritoneal dialysis (CAPD). Her physician ordered epoetin alfa (Procrit) 150 units/kg to be given subcutaneously three times a week. Today the client weighs 80 kg.

a.   How many units of Procrit should you give to this client? Show your work below. Have another student, or your instructor, check your work for feedback.

b.   The Procrit vial is labeled as 10,000 units/mL. How much medication in milliliters will deliver the required units to the client? Show your work below.

c.   Administer the medication to the client and document your action.

d.   What laboratory test values should you monitor to determine if the medication has been effective?

Critical Thinking Activity 18-1-4

A middle-aged woman diagnosed with relapsing-remitting multiple sclerosis is prescribed to take interferon beta-1b recombinant (Betaseron) 9.6 million IU (0.3 mg) SC. As the office nurse, you need to teach her how to self-administer this drug.

a.   To mix the medication in the single-dose vial, 1.2 mL of diluent is needed. Prepare the medication now.

b.   How much of the medication should you teach the client to draw up into the syringe?

c.   Provide health teaching for the client and show her how to give a subcutaneous injection.

Critical Thinking Activity 18-1-5

You are working in an urban child wellness clinic. The nurse practitioner asks you to administer a mumps skin test antigen (MSTA) to a 7-year old child.

a.   What route should be used to ensure an accurate skin test result?

b.   Demonstrate this procedure on the child. Give 0.1 mL.

c.   What is the purpose of skin testing? What other skin tests are available?

Learning Objectives

The learner is expected to:

1. Demonstrate how to administer intramuscular medications, including the Z-tract method.

2. Calculate medication dosing for adults.

3. Identify appropriate laboratory test values that should be monitored for clients receiving selected medications.

4. Document medication administration on the appropriate medical records.

5. Explain the purpose of selected medications.

Critical Thinking Skill Practice and Validation

• Analysis

• Explanation

• Evaluation

• Self-regulation

Critical Thinking Activity 18-2-1

A young obese adult complains of acute pain and has an order for butorphanol (Stadol) 3 mg IM Q4H PRN. You prepare to give the medication.

a.   The vial of Stadol is labeled as 2 mg/mL. How much of the drug should you administer? Show your work below. Have another student, or your instructor, check your work for feedback.

b.   Administer the drug to the client. Will your procedure or site selection vary because the client is obese? Why or why not?

Critical Thinking Activity 18-2-2

One of your young adult clients in the nursing home is diagnosed with severe iron deficiency anemia. The physician orders iron dextran (DexFerum) 100 mg QD IM X 5 days. A test dose resulted in no adverse reaction.

a.   Demonstrate how to give this medication. Remember that intramuscular iron is very irritating to body tissues.

b.   What laboratory test values should you monitor to determine if the drug is effective and why?

c.   What are common side/adverse effects of IM iron?

Critical Thinking Activity 18-2-3

You are caring for a middle-aged woman following an abdominal hysterectomy and bilateral salpingo-oophorectomy (BSO). The client complains of severe incisional pain. The surgeon ordered meperidine (Demerol) 100 mg with hydroxyzine HCl (Vistaril) 25 mg IM Q3-4H PRN for pain. You prepare to give the medication.

a.   Why is Vistaril ordered in combination with Demerol for this client?

b.   What physical assessment should you perform before giving the drug?

c.   When you check the available Demerol, you find that 100 mg is packaged in a prefilled syringe. The Vistaril comes in a vial labeled 50 mg/mL. How much Vistaril will you administer? Show your work below.

d.   Demonstrate how you should mix these medications and administer the injection to your client. Document your medication administration on the appropriate medical records.

Learning Objectives

The student is expected to:

1. Demonstrate how to give intravenous (IV) push medications via a saline lok.

2. Identify desired outcomes for selected IV medications.

3. Calculate IV medication dosing for infants.

4. Calculate IV medication dosing for adults.

5. Describe adverse effects of selected IV medications.

6. Demonstrate and document the administration of medications mixed with large-volume IV fluids.

7. Add medication to a patient-controlled analgesia (PCA) medication delivery system and document care of the client receiving PCA.

8. Define common terms associated with parenteral medications.

Critical Thinking Skill Practice and Validation

*   Interpretation

*   Analysis

*   Explanation

*   Evaluation

*   Inference

*   Self-regulation

Critical Thinking Activity 18-3-1

An older adult presents in the ED with acute congestive heart failure (CHF) and pulmonary edema. She has bilateral crackles in her lower lobes and dyspnea at rest. The physician orders furosemide (Lasix) 40 mg IV push (IVP) via her saline lok. The vial is labeled as 10 mg/mL.

a.   How much Lasix should you give her in milliliters? Show your work below. Have another student, or your instructor, check your work for feedback.

b.   What desired effect is expected from the drug and when might you expect it? What physical assessment findings will show that the effect has been achieved?

c.   Demonstrate how to give this medication via a saline lok.

d.   What laboratory test values should you monitor before and after medication administration?

Critical Thinking Activity 18-3-2

A 3-week old infant is admitted to the pediatric unit with septicemia. She currently weighs 10.6 lb. The physician orders cefotaxime sodium (Claforan) 50 mg/kg IV Q8H.

a.   How much medication in mg should you give the child every 8 hours? Show your work below. Have another student, or your instructor, check your work for feedback.

b.   Demonstrate how to give the IV medication for the infant using either a piggyback or burette method. Use a needleless system if one is available.

c.   What adverse effects should you monitor for?

Critical Thinking Activity 18-3-3

An adult client is having surgery for bladder cancer this morning and has an order for gentamicin sulfate 80 mg IVPB in 100 mL NS to be given preoperatively.

a.   Why is the client receiving this medication prior to surgery?

b.   At what rate should you set the IV pump to deliver this IV piggyback medication and why?

c.   What side/adverse effects are common with this medication?

d.   Demonstrate how to administer this medication using the IVPB method. (The client has a 1000 mL bag of 5%D/0.45NS running at 133 mL/hr.) Use a needleless system if one is available.

Critical Thinking Activity 18-3-4

A young adult client has an order for 1000 mL 5%D/NS with 60 mEq KCl to run at 125 mL/hr postoperatively.

a. How many mEq of KCl will be delivered at this IV rate? Show your work below. Have another student, or your instructor, check for feedback.

b. Demonstrate hanging a new bag of the prescribed IV solution. Should this IV solution be regulated by an infusion pump? Why or why not?

c. On the unit you have a 500 mL bag of 5%D/NS premixed with 40 mEq KCl. Should you use this bag? Why or why not?

d. What are the clinical manifestations of hyperkalemia?

Critical Thinking Activity 18-3-5

A young adult is receiving continuous heparin for deep vein thrombosis (DVT) in her left thigh. The physician ordered 1800 units per hour continuous IV. The pharmacy sends up the premixed bag of medication for this infusion.

a. Should a continuous heparin infusion be controlled by an electronic pump? Why or why not?

b. The first bag is labeled as "25,000 units in 500 mL 0.45% NS. Run at 41 mL/hr." Will this rate deliver the prescribed dose? Show your work below. Have another student, or your instructor, check your work for feedback.

c. What is the antidote for heparin?

d. What physical assessment should you perform and document while the client is receiving heparin?

Critical Thinking 18-3-6

A young adult returns from the PACU following a total thyroidectomy for thyroid cancer. She has a PCA pump for continuous and intermittent dosing of morphine sulfate for acute postoperative pain. When she is admitted to your unit, you perform a complete postoperative assessment and review of her surgeon's orders.

a.   What position should the client be placed in and why?

b.   The order for morphine indicates that the client should receive a continuous infusion of 0.5 mg/hr and can use the PCA to deliver an additional 8 mg over a 4-hour period if needed. The lockout interval is 15 minutes. How many mg can she self-administer with each PCA bolus? Show your work below. Have another student, or your instructor, check your work for feedback.

c.   What physical assessment should you perform and document at least every 4 hours and why?

d.   If the client uses the PCA bolus 5 times in 4 hours, what is the TOTAL
     amount of morphine that she received?

e.   Demonstrate adding a 30-mL morphine vial labeled 1 mg/mL. Document
     this action on the appropriate PCA flow sheet, if available.

f.   What should you do if the client becomes dizzy, hypotensive and/or has a
     respiratory rate of less than 10 per minute?

Critical Thinking Activity 18-3-7

An older client returns from PACU with an epidural catheter in place for analgesia for 24 hours postoperatively. When you check the surgeon's orders, you note that the client is receiving continuous fentanyl controlled by an epidural infusion pump. When you assess the client on admission to the unit, you find that she is a 2 on a 0 to 10 pain scale.

a.   What can you conclude about the client's current level of pain?

b.   When you check the client an hour later, you find that her respiratory rate has decreased to 6 and the client is difficult to arouse. You give her Narcan 0.2 mg IVP per hospital policy and notify the anesthesiologist. Demonstrate this procedure now and document it. What are the desired outcomes of this action?

c.   What would you expect her level of pain to be after administering the Narcan? Why?

Review of Terms 18-3-8

Match the term in the left column with its definition from the right column.

___1. Subcutaneous

___2. Intradermal

___3. Intramuscular

___4. Z- tract method

___5. Intravenous

___6. IV piggyback (IVPB)

___7. IV push (IVP)

___8. Patient-controlled analgesia (PCA)

___9. Opioid

___10. Epidural

A. Entered into the vein

B. Type of narcotic analgesia

C. Into the dermis of the skin

D. Method where client can self-medicate opioids and other drugs

E. Deep IM method used for irritating medications

F. Into the space outside the dura mater

G. Into the muscle

H. Delivery of medication directly into the vein

I. Into the fatty tissue

J. Delivery of diluted medication through the port of a main IV line

Hadaway, L.C. (2001). How to safeguard delivery of high-alert IV drugs. *Nursing2001, 31*(2), pp. 36-41.

This excellent review article describes the precautions that are needed when administering IV drugs such as potassium, insulin, heparin and dopamine. Medication dosing and delivery are among many nursing considerations that the author discusses. A quiz is found at the end of the article.

Jew, R.K., Gordin, P., & Lengetti, E. (1997). Clinical implications of IV drug administration in infants and children. *Critical Care Nurse, 17*(4), pp. 62-70.

The authors discuss the challenge of IV medication administration in children and precautions that are needed for that group when compared to adults. Nursing implications are described and suggestions for anticipated problems are described.

Skokal, W. (2000). IV push at home? *RN, 63*(10), pp. 26-29.

This article discusses the increasing trend for IV push medication to be given by home care nurses and others trained in the procedure. As hospitals discharge clients early from acute care, continued client care at home may require the use of IV medications.

Woods, M. (2000). Advanced skills update: Patient-controlled analgesia. *Professional Nurse, 15*(6), pp. 404-405.

This brief article reviews the procedure and documentation for patient-controlled analgesia (PCA). The author describes both the continuous and bolus functions of the PCA pumps.

UNIT 19. PERIPHERAL INTRAVENOUS (IV) THERAPY

19-1.　Initiation of Peripheral Therapy

19-2.　Care and Maintenance of Peripheral IV Therapy

Suggested Readings

19-1. INITIATION OF PERIPHERAL THERAPY

Learning Objectives

The learner is expected to:

1. Identify the physical assessment that is needed prior to starting peripheral IV therapy.

2. Calculate IV fluid flow rates for adults and children.

3. Demonstrate how to insert an over-the-needle catheter.

4. Apply an IV site dressing for a peripheral IV.

5. Explain what factors can influence IV fluid flow rate.

Critical Thinking Skill Practice and Validation

- Analysis

- Explanation

- Inference

- Self-regulation

Critical Thinking Activity 19-1-1

An alert and oriented older adult is admitted to your hospital unit with an order to start an IV of 5%D/0.2% to run continuously at 100 mL/hr. She most likely will have abdominal surgery later in the day. When you review her history, you note that she has Type II diabetes mellitus and asthma, which is controlled by chronic steroid therapy (Prednisone).

a.   What physical assessment should you perform before starting her IV therapy and why?

b.   Demonstrate how to initiate peripheral IV therapy using an over-the-needle catheter. Cover the site with a transparent dressing.

c.   How should your IV insertion procedure vary based on this client's assessment?

d.	There are no infusion pumps available at this time on the unit. How many drops per minute (gtts/min) will be needed to deliver 100 mL/min? Show your work below. Have another student, or your instructor, check your work for feedback.

e.	If the client becomes restless, disoriented and acutely confused, what action should you take, if any?

Critical Thinking Activity 19-1-2

When you later check on the client in Critical Thinking Activity 19-1-1, you notice that only 100 mL of her IV fluids have infused during the past two hours. The IV was inserted into her left forearm.

a.   What possible factors could explain why the client did not receive the correct amount of fluid?

b.   What physical assessment should you perform at this time?

c.   What action should you take to ensure that the client will receive an accurate amount of IV fluids?

Critical Thinking Activity 19-1-3

A 4-year old is admitted to the pediatric unit with a respiratory infection and is receiving IV fluids and antibiotics. The drop factor for the continuous IV peripheral set is 60 gtts/mL

a.   If the IV fluid is running at 50 mL/hour, what flow rate (in gtts/min) is being delivered? Show your work below.

b.   The child complains to you that his arm hurts while he is receiving the IV antibiotic. What action should you take at this time?

c.   If the IV becomes dislodged, how does IV insertion differ for a young child when compared to IV insertion for an adult?

Learning Objectives

The learner is expected to:

1.   Explain the difference between partial and total parenteral nutrition (PPN and TPN).

2.   Describe the care required for a client who has PPN.

3.   Demonstrate how to discontinue a peripheral IV line.

4.   Change an IV tubing set and IV bag using sterile technique.

5.   Perform and document assessments for clients receiving blood transfusions.

6.   Administer a blood transfusion.

7.   Convert a continuous peripheral IV to an intermittent saline/heparin lok.

Critical Thinking Skill Practice and Validation

- Explanation

- Self-regulation

- Analysis

- Inference

Critical Thinking Activity 19-2-1

A middle-aged adult is receiving partial parenteral nutrition (PPN) through a peripheral line for pancreatitis at a local nursing home. As his nurse, you perform an assessment and check on his PPN.

a.   How will you determine if the PPN is effective? How is it different from TPN? What assessments should you perform for the client related to PPN?

b.   The client's PPN bag is almost empty and the new bag is not yet available. What should you do? Demonstrate how to add a new bag to the system.

c.   The IV tubing needs to be changed today. Demonstrate how to change the tubing for this client's PPN administration.

d.   When you check the client's IV site, you note that it is reddened and warm. Demonstrate how to discontinue the IV now.

e.   Write a note below to document your actions during this activity. Have another student, or your instructor, check your note for feedback.

Critical Thinking Activity 19-2-2

One day after having a total hip replacement, a middle-aged adult needs to receive an autologous blood transfusion. Her hemoglobin and hematocrit have decreased dramatically since surgery. She has 5%D/NS running at 75 mL/hr.

a.   Can you **delegate** any part of this action to unlicensed assistive personnel? If so, what can you ask them to do?

b.   When you receive the blood from the laboratory, what do you need to check?

c.   What equipment and supplies will you need to start the transfusion?

d.   Demonstrate how to hang the blood. What assessments will you need to perform during blood administration?

e.   About an hour after the blood transfusion is started, the client's temperature increases to 101 degrees F. The client complains that she "feels hot" and then has chills. What should you do first and why?

f.   Write a note below to describe this event and your interventions. Have another student, or your instructor, check your note for feedback.

g.   After the blood transfusion, convert the peripheral IV into a saline/heparin lok (INT).

SUGGESTED READINGS

Dougherty, L. (2000). Intravenous infusions: Calculating rates. *Nursing Times, 96*(10), pp. 51-52.

The author reviews the basics of how to calculate drip rates when electronic devices are not available. Several methods are reviewed to determine how many drops per minute deliver the prescribed IV fluid amount.

Duck, S. (1997). Neonatal intravenous nursing. *Journal of Intravenous Nursing, 20*(3), 121-128.

This article describes the special need of neonates who require intravenous therapy. Site selection, precautions, and nursing implications are discussed. Complications—how to prevent them, monitor for them and detect them early— are also outlined.

Williams, C. & Lefever, J. (2000). Reducing the user error with infusion pumps. *Professional Nurse, 15*(6), pp. 382-384.

The authors discuss how to properly use electronic infusion pumps and focus on how to reduce errors, such as incorrect settings for flow rates. They disprove the myth that infusion pumps prevent all errors related to intravenous flow rates.

UNIT 20. CENTRAL INTRAVENOUS (IV) THERAPY

20-1. Care and Maintenance of Central IV Therapy

20-2. Special Procedures Related to Central IV Therapy

Suggested Readings

20-1. CARE AND MAINTENANCE OF CENTRAL IV THERAPY

Learning Objectives

The learner is expected to:

1. Describe the purpose and special care related to central IV therapy.

2. Explain complications of central IV therapy.

3. Identify the advantages of a peripherally-inserted central catheter (PICC).

4. Demonstrate how to access an implanted infusion port, if available.

5. Define common terms associated with central IV therapy.

Critical Thinking Skill Practice and Validation

- Explanation

- Analysis

- Inference

- Evaluation

Critical Thinking Activity 20-1-1

A severely undernourished and neglected 13-year old boy is admitted to the hospital and placed on total parenteral nutrition (TPN). He is developmentally disabled.

a.   What are the desired outcomes for the child related to nutritional health?

b.   What are the advantages of a central line when compared to a peripheral line?

c.   What assessments are required for the client related to central IV therapy and TPN?

d.   What complications are associated with central IV therapy and why?

Critical Thinking Activity 20-1-2

A young adult client is recovering from extensive trauma as a result of a motor vehicle accident. The client has developed chronic osteomyelitis and needs many months of antibiotic therapy via a central line. He is discharged to home where his mother and wife will provide his care. You are the nurse who will teach the family how to be effective caregivers.

a.   Demonstrate how the family should administer the appropriate IV minibags.

b.   The home care nurse visits twice a week to check on the client and his family. During the third week, the client's wife complains that the last minibag of medication infused very slowly, even after the line was flushed. The nurse assesses the central catheter and decides to discontinue the line. What is the procedure for removing a central catheter? Is removal of a central line within the scope of nursing practice? What options does the nurse have to regain an IV access for the antibiotic therapy?

c.   How is a PICC different from a Hickman or Groshong central catheter?

d.   What is an implanted infusion port and how does it differ from a Hickman or Groshong central catheter?

e.   If available, demonstrate how to access an implanted port.

20-2. SPECIAL PROCEDURES RELATED TO CENTRAL IV THERAPY

Learning Objectives

The learner is expected to:

1. Explain special precautions needed for clients receiving chemotherapy.

2. Demonstrate how to draw blood from a central IV catheter.

3. Demonstrate how to change a central line dressing.

Critical Thinking Skill Practice and Validation

- Explanation

- Analysis

- Inference

Critical Thinking Activity 20-2-1

A middle-aged client has lymphoma and is receiving multiple chemotherapeutic medications via a central IV line. She lives at home with her husband and son, and goes to the Ambulatory Infusion Center in a local hospital three days a week. She has frequent blood tests to monitor for adverse effects of chemotherapy. You are a nurse working at the center.

a.   What special precautions are needed for chemotherapy administration?

b.   What is extravasation? How is it avoided and how is it treated if it occurs?

Critical Thinking Activity 20-2-2

You explain the central line care needed for the client in Critical Thinking Activity 20-2-1 as part of your health teaching.

a.   Explain and demonstrate how to draw blood from her double-lumen line for a CBC.

b.   Why is a CBC frequently performed for clients receiving chemotherapy?

c.   Demonstrate how to change her central line dressing and explain the rationale for each step.

Review of Terms 20-2-3

Match the term in the left column with its definition from the right column.

___1. Extravasation

A. A central venous access device placed through an arm vein

___2. Huber needle

B. The presence of air in the sub-cutaneous tissue

___3. Peripherally-inserted central catheter (PICC)

C. Subcutaneously implanted plastic or metal case that provides venous access

___4. Tunneled catheter

D. IV fluid leakage into soft tissues

___5. Infusion port

E. Right-angled or straight non-coring needle used for ports

___6. Central venous access device (CVAD)

F. Any catheter or device placed into the internal jugular or sub-clavian vein

___7. Total parenteral nutrition (TPN)

G. Leakage of highly toxic irritants into soft tissue

___8. Air embolism

H. IV solution that contains all nutrients that the body needs

___9. Infiltration

I. Obstruction of a blood vessel caused by an air bubble

___10. Subcutaneous emphysema

J. A single-, double- or triple-lumen catheter, inserted into a central vein through sub-cutaneous tissue and exiting on the chest or abdomen

SUGGESTED READINGS

Carlson, K.R. (1999). Correct utilization and management of peripherally inserted central catheters. *Journal of Intravenous Nursing, 22*(Suppl), S46-50.

This supplement to the journal outlines the appropriate indications for use of PICCs. It also describes the care that is required to ensure that the PICC functions properly and ways to minimize complications.

Drewett, S.R. (2000). Complications of central venous catheters: Nursing care. *British Journal of Nursing, 9*(8), 466-468, 470-478.

The author describes the risks and complications commonly associated with the use of invasive central IV therapy. The devices that are used, as well as the solutions that are delivered through central lines, make clients vulnerable to potentially life-threatening health problems, such as infection and air embolism.

Schmid, M.W. (2000). Risks and complications of peripherally and centrally inserted intravenous catheters. *Critical Care Nursing Clinics of North America, 12*(2), pp. 165-174.

This article discussed common risks at which clients are placed when they require either peripheral or central IV therapy. Both types of therapy are invasive procedures that increase risk of infection and other potentially life-threatening complications. Nurses need to observe for these complications and take measures, when possible, to prevent them.

UNIT 21. PRIORITY SETTING SKILLS

21-1. Individual Adult Client Care

21-2. Managing a Group of Adult Clients

21-1. INDIVIDUAL ADULT CLIENT CARE

Learning Objectives

The learner is expected to:

1.   Prioritize care for a newly admitted adult client.

2.   Identify the client's primary nursing diagnoses / collaborative problems.

3.   Identify expected outcomes for the client.

4.   Explain the rationale for prioritizing the client's care.

Critical Thinking Skill Practice and Validation

- Explanation

- Analysis

- Inference

- Evaluation

- Interpretation

- Self-regulation

Critical Thinking Activity 21-1-1**

An 89-year old diabetic is admitted to your medical-surgical unit with hyperglycemia (BS=480) from the ED. The medication administration record (MAR) states that insulin was given, but does not include the time or dosage. The client lives at home alone and was diagnosed with an upper respiratory infection two days ago. The physician's orders are:

Admitting DX: Uncontrolled diabetes, pneumonia
Diet: No added sugar
Activity: BRP
VS Q 4H
Pulse oximetry Q 8H and PRN
Allergies: Sulfa drugs
Insert Foley catheter to SD; obtain urine for C & S
Meds:

      10u Humulin R/20u Humulin N SC Q AM AC breakfast
      Erythromycin 500 mg BID
      Ativan 1-2 mg IM Q 8H PRN
      TB Mantoux ID today

Your initial assessment findings include VS 99-88(reg)-20, 154/88. He is alert and oriented to person only. His skin is warm and dry and he complains of thirst. His face is flushed and he is restless and fidgety. He states that he has not eaten today. The client's daughter is concerned about his change in health and is seated at his bedside.

a.   Prioritize your care for this client, including a comprehensive assessment. Pretend that a fellow student or your instructor is the daughter.

b.   Provide medications and treatments in the appropriate order and explain your rationale.

c.   When you take the client's FSBS again, you note that it is now 240. What is the significance of this finding?

d.   What other interventions might the client need for which you need an order and why?

Critical Thinking Activity 21-1-2**

A young Asian American client has been hospitalized for two days after being stabbed in the chest. He has posterior chest tubes connected to a Pleur-Evac chest drainage system. A policeman is stationed outside the room. At 7AM, the night nurse reported that the client had a restless night. His chest drainage was 15 mL; VS were 99-90-22, 128/74. His pulse ox was 95%. The client's IV needs to be restarted because he just pulled it out.

a.   What other assessment data do you need?

b.   Why do you need the additional information in a. above?

The physician's orders include:
VS Q 4H
Ambulate with assist
Oxygen at 2-3L via NC
Pulse ox Q 4H
Chest tube to low continuous suction
IV 1000 mL 5%D/ 1/2 NS Q 12 H
IVPB cefazolin 1 g Q 6H
Colace 100 mg PO QD
Chest x-ray today
ABG today
Soft diet

The history states that the client was arrested for attempted rape at a residence, and the mother of the family allegedly defended herself with a kitchen knife, causing the chest wound. The client will be discharged to the county jail until the trial date.

Your 8AM assessment includes VS 99^8 - 92-26, 140/90. The client continues to be restless, c/o dyspnea, and is anxious. He has bilateral lower lobe crackles and his pulse ox is now 88% after he pulled off his nasal cannula.

c.   What should your priority actions be at this time and why?

d.   At 9AM, the client complains of pain. After receiving an order for Demerol 75 mg IM Q3-4 H PRN, you prepare to get the medication. While the client turns over to receive his IM Demerol, the chest tube becomes dislodged. What should you do at this time and why?

Cases are courtesy of Arlene H. Morris, MSN, RN, Instructor of Nursing at Auburn University Montgomery School of Nursing in Montgomery, Alabama.

21-2. MANAGING A GROUP OF ADULT CLIENTS

Learning Objectives

The learner is expected to:

1. Prioritize care for a select group of adult clients.

2. Provide rationale for prioritization of care.

3. Determine which part of nursing care can be delegated to unlicensed assistive personnel.

Critical Thinking Skill Practice and Validation

- Analysis

- Interpretation

- Inference

- Explanation

Critical Thinking Activity 21-2-1

You are assigned to care for 5 clients on a busy medical-surgical unit. The following information is given in report at 3PM:

234A Older client is in the OR for a BK amputation due to PVD and DM; expected back at 4PM

234B Middle-aged client is recovering from colon resection surgery with colostomy. Had surgery yesterday and got OOB for the first time this AM. Was dizzy and had to be put back to bed in 5 minutes. PCA Demerol infusing continuously and client has used bolus 3 times during the last 8 hours.

236 Young client continues on contact isolation for infected foot surgery, possible osteomyelitis. Receiving antibiotics and c/o boredom in the hospital. Wants to go home with IV therapy.

237A Older client admitted today from a local nursing home with abdominal pain. Has Alzheimer's disease and h/o CHF, stroke, CAD. Poor appetite and dehydrated. Receiving continuous IV therapy, but has pulled the catheter out twice so far today. Has no family in the area.

237B Older client returned from OR three hours ago with abdominal hysterectomy. Alert and oriented, dressing dry and intact, IV at KVO rate until client voids and takes more fluids. No c/o N/V. Pain being controlled with PCA morphine.

a. Is there additional information that you might need from report on any of these clients? If so, what do you need to know and why?

b. Which client would you check on first and why?

Critical Thinking Activity 21-2-2

You assign a PCA (Patient Care Associate) to work with you to provide client care for the clients in Critical Thinking Activity 21-2-1. She is also helping another nurse who has five clients in her group.

a.   What care could you delegate to an unlicensed nursing staff member and why?

b.   You ask the PCA to help you change the client in 237A because she is incontinent. The PCA tells you that she is busy helping the other nurse to whom she has been assigned. What should you do?